Osteoporosis - Pathophysiology, Diagnosis, Management and Therapy

Edited by Rupesh K. Srivastava

Published in London, United Kingdom

Osteoporosis - Pathophysiology, Diagnosis, Management and Therapy
http://dx.doi.org/10.5772/intechopen.111138
Edited by Rupesh K. Srivastava

Contributors
Pengguo Gou, Feng Chang, Vardhan Pol, Taranjeet Kaur, Asha Bhardwaj, Leena Sapra, Sumedha Yadav, Rupesh K. Srivastava, Riya Mukherjee, Chung-Ming Chang, Ramendra Pati Pandey, Maxuel Fidelis de Padua Almeida, Guilherme Donadel, Mariana Dalmagro, Gabriel Maciel, Gabriela Zanuto de Lima, Marcia Alessandra Arantes Marques, Salviano Tramontin Bellettini, Ezilda Jacomassi, Giuliana Zardeto, Emerson Luiz Botelho Lourenço, Daniela de Cassia Faglioni Boleta Ceranto, Sayantee Hazra, Shagnik Chattopadhyay, Ritobrata Goswami

First published in London, United Kingdom, 2024 by IntechOpen
IntechOpen is the global imprint of INTECHOPEN LIMITED, registered in England and Wales, registration number: 11086078, 5 Princes Gate Court, London, SW7 2QJ, United Kingdom

British Library Cataloguing-in-Publication Data
A catalogue record for this book is available from the British Library

Additional hard and PDF copies can be obtained from orders@intechopen.com

Osteoporosis - Pathophysiology, Diagnosis, Management and Therapy
Edited by Rupesh K. Srivastava
p. cm.
Print ISBN 978-0-85466-080-3
Online ISBN 978-0-85466-079-7
eBook (PDF) ISBN 978-0-85466-081-0

For EU product safety concerns:
IN TECH d.o.o., Prolaz Marije Krucifikse Kozulić 3, 51000 Rijeka, Croatia,
info@intechopen.com or visit our website at intechopen.com.

Meet the editor

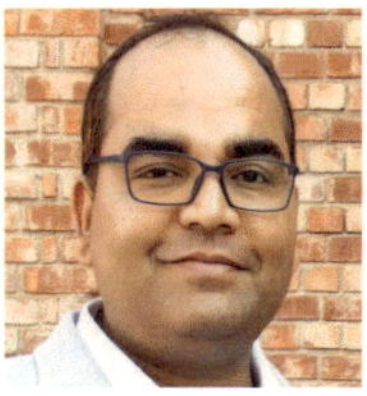

Dr. Rupesh K. Srivastava is an associate professor in the Department of Biotechnology, All India Institute of Medical Sciences (AIIMS), New Delhi, India. He received his a Ph.D. from the National Centre of Cell Sciences (NCCS), Pune, India in 2011. He completed his postdoctoral research at Columbia University Medical Centre (CUMC), NY, USA, and Roswell Park Cancer Institute (RPCI), Buffalo, New York, USA. He is an immunologist and has contributed to the discovery of a novel field of biology called "immunoporosis" by elucidating the critical involvement of the immune system in the pathophysiology of osteoporosis. His long-term vision is to develop innovative and effective immunotherapeutic approaches for the treatment and management of osteoporosis by taking advantage of the role of different immune cells in its pathophysiology.

Contents

Preface

This book provides a comprehensive review of osteoporosis. Osteoporosis is a skeletal disorder that affects the microarchitecture and mineralization of bone, reduces bone strength, and lowers bone mineral density (BMD). Osteoporosis poses a serious threat to the public healthcare system. It is a composite and complex disease because multiple molecular culprits work together to contribute to its emergence and progression. Fractures due to osteoporosis can raise overall healthcare expenses, discomfort, disability, and mortality. Therefore, management of osteoporosis and its associated consequences is essential for enhancing quality of life and lessening the financial strain on the healthcare system. As scientists learn more about the underlying mechanisms of osteoporosis, significant therapeutic advancements in treating the condition have been made in recent years.

Osteoporosis – Pathophysiology, Diagnosis, Management and Therapy compiles perceptive information on the most recent findings, opinions, and reviews in osteoporosis from writers, scientists, and medical professionals worldwide. This compilation represents a genuine attempt to compile inputs from globally recognized academicians, researchers, and clinicians to identify the cellular and molecular offenders that contribute to the agony and suffering experienced by those with osteoporosis.

This volume is comprised of five chapters. Chapter 1, "Drug Therapeutics of Osteoporosis, Vertebral Fracture and Nonunion", elaborates on the treatment of osteoporosis, osteoporotic vertebral compression fractures (OVCFs), and nonunion. Nearly half of all osteoporotic fractures are OVCFs, the most prevalent type of single-fragility fracture. Recent findings have brought attention to the extensive communication network that exists between the immune system and bone in the maintenance of bone homeostasis. Furthermore, most of the first-line therapies for osteoporosis can modulate the immune system and thereby prevent bone resorption by regulating the immune system. Chapter 2, "Targeting "Immunoporosis" as a Novel Concept of Immunotherapy in the Management and Treatment of Osteoporosis", and Chapter 3, "Immunology and Osteoporosis: A New Frontier in Treatment", provide insights into the crucial role of the immune system in the pathophysiology of osteoporosis (i.e., immunoporosis) along with several novel immunomodulatory strategies that can be exploited for its management and treatment. Chapter 4, "Evaluation of *Plinia cauliflora* Effect in the Prevention of Osteoporosis in Ovariectomized Rats", evaluates the effect of the extract of herbal plant *Plinia cauliflora* in the prevention of osteoporosis in ovariectomized rats. Chapter 5, "Immunomodulation of Bone Remodeling in Osteoporosis", discusses the complex interplay between the immune system, associated cytokines, and bone remodeling.

I am grateful to all the researchers and clinicians for their outstanding contributions. I extend my heartfelt gratitude to the staff at IntechOpen, especially Publishing Process Manager Zrinka Tomicic, for their gracious assistance and support throughout the publication process.

We hope that readers will find this book to be enjoyable to read and a valuable source of information for their work.

Happy Reading!

Rupesh K. Srivastava
Associate Professor,
Department of Biotechnology,
All India Institute of Medical Sciences (AIIMS),
New Delhi, India

Chapter 1

Drug Therapeutics of Osteoporosis, Vertebral Fracture and Nonunion

Pengguo Gou and Feng Chang

Abstract

Osteoporosis management is effective in decreasing vertebral fracture risk. The assessment of vertebral fracture risk is used to identify patients with high fracture risk for anti-osteoporotic treatment, especially for those who have not yet fractured. Several pharmacological agents are available to lower vertebral fracture risk by reducing bone resorption or/and stimulating bone formation. Aside from surgical treatment for fresh vertebral fracture or fracture nonunion in elderly patients, recent studies indicated that management of osteoporosis plays a vital role in boosting vertebral fracture union, preventing progressive vertebral collapse and decreasing the refracture risk. In this chapter, we focus on the treatment of osteoporosis, acute vertebral fractures and nonunion, as well as the evaluation of clinical efficacy by bone quality and bone turnover markers after treatment.

Keywords: osteoporosis, spine, vertebral fracture, drug therapies, anti-resorptive treatment, anabolic treatment

1. Introduction

Osteoporosis (OP), an age-related metabolic bone disease characterized by low bone mass and microarchitectural deterioration of bone tissue, increases the risk of fractures in the elderly population [1]. The prevalence of osteoporosis over the age of 50 years is 23% in men and 7% in women. It is emerging as a serious public health problem worldwide and brings severe challenges to the global health and social service sector because of aging of the population, especially in developing countries [2].

Osteoporotic vertebral compression fractures (OVCFs), the most common single fragility fractures, account for almost 50% of all osteoporotic fractures [3]. OVCFs are the most common type of osteoporotic fractures and often occur in the absence of trauma or following a low-energy trauma (a fall from a standing height or less) [4–6]. Worldwide, the incidence of OVCFs was 30–50% of people over age 50 and increased with age in both men and women [3, 7]. Acute OVCF patients commonly suffer from significant and long-lasting back pain, substantially impacting the patients' Health-related quality of life (HRQoL) [8–12]. Magnetic resonance imaging (MRI) features are crucial to achieving an accurate and early diagnosis, on which the bone marrow signals displayed hypointensity on T1-weighted and hyperintensity on T2-weighted and fat-suppressed sequences within a deformed vertebral body [13–15]. OVCFs were acute if the interval between the trauma or symptom onset and MRI was less than 2 weeks [16, 17]. It is also a major risk factor to subsequent refractures, which are also called vertebral fracture cascade [18, 19]. In the first year after an OVCF, risks of refractures increase by 4–7 times [20, 21]. The progressive loss of anterior height leads to spinal kyphotic deformities and imposes more stress on the anterior spinal column, increasing the risk of new OVCFs [22]. In addition, kyphotic deformity also disrupts body balance, resulting in an increased risk of falls and other fractures [22].

Not all OVCFs could heal following conservative treatment. Once nonunion occurs, the intractable back pain and even neurological deficits further decrease the HRQoL [23, 24]. In addition to increased morbidity and mortality, it imposes a significant economic burden on the public health systems worldwide and patient families [2, 23, 25].

The anti-osteoporosis (anti-OP) management to prevent OVCFs is one of the most important objectives, a chronic and long-term condition even requiring lifelong management [26]. The advice in this passage provides a framework for healthcare professionals. The detailed treatment plans should be based on the individual situations in clinical practice.

2. Risk assessment of OVCFs

2.1 Background

Osteoporosis is a significant risk factor for OVCFs. In postmenopausal women and men aged more than 50 years, the risk factors of OVCFs are assessed to determine whether anti-OP therapy is needed to reduce the fracture risks. If at high risk of fracture, the anti-OP to prevent subsequent fractures is advised as early as possible. Fractures are common in severe osteoporosis patients, particularly among older women. Generally, anti-OP therapy is advised in patients having a bone mineral density (BMD) T-score of −2.5 or less, a history of spine or hip fracture or a Fracture Risk Assessment Tool (FRAX) score indicating increased fracture risk [16, 27]. In addition, the refracture risk is multiplied following the initial fracture in OVCF patients, indicating the need for anti-OP therapy to prevent subsequent fractures [20, 28].

Several fracture risk assessment tools, including the BMD, FRAX, QFracture and Garvan fracture risk calculator, have been developed to estimate the fracture risk in OP patients. Unfortunately, fracture risk prediction remains an imprecise science.

2.2 BMD

Bone mineral density could be an option for the prediction of OVCFs risk. In clinical practice, BMD measured with dual-energy X-ray absorptiometry (DXA) is closely related to OVCFs risk and incorporated in most risk assessment paradigms. Each 1-standard deviation (1-SD) reduction is associated with an increased fracture risk of 1.5–2-fold. However, the BMD is not sensitive in the assessment of osteoporosis. OVCFs may occur in individuals with a BMD above this threshold (T-score > −2.5), reflecting the other factors contributing to fracture risk [29, 30]. Such clinical risk factors as age, sex, smoking, weight loss and glucocorticoid use have been noted with OVCFs risk and included in the risk assessment, even in the absence of BMD.

2.3 FRAX

Fracture Risk Assessment score (http://www.shef.ac.uk/FRAX), the most widely used fracture risk assessment tool, allows an accurate assessment of 10-year OVCFs risk without BMD T-score and could help to make treatment decisions [31]. Its significant feature is that it can be directly calibrated to fracture incidence rates in the target population and considers death a competing risk. Most clinical practice guidelines incorporated it for assessing the OVCFs risk in many countries. High fracture risk patients are recommended anti-OP treatment, especially for those who have not yet sustained an OVCF. Treatment is unnecessary for those patients with very low fracture risk, and an intermediate group of patients undergoes BMD testing to refine their fracture risk. Therefore, an osteopenic individual with a BMD T-score of −2.5 to −1.0 but with high OVCF risk should be administered anti-OP therapy.

However, the FRAX was only used in patients with a BMD T-score ≤ −1.0 and without anti-OP treatment. Neither follow-up patients nor those patients treated for osteoporosis or osteopenia are appropriate for taking up this risk assessment tool. In addition, such limitations, including the inability to identify the imminent fracture risk, underestimated OVCFs risk in diabetic patients, fracture risk stratification for the exposure of different dose glucocorticoids and fall risk, have not been settled [32, 33].

It is important to emphasize that FRAX is not a substitute for BMD, which can be reserved for osteoporosis diagnosis.

2.4 QFracture

QFracture (www.qfracture.org), primarily applicable to the UK population, could predict the 1–10-year OVCFs, independent of BMD in primary care. Like the FRAX, it includes several causes of osteoporosis, such as a history of smoking, alcohol, corticosteroid use, parental history of osteoporosis and several secondary causes of osteoporosis. Besides, a history of falls was included, utilizing a large number of clinical risk factors. A feature of QFracture is that it contains more questions and does not accommodate the inclusion of BMD for assessing fracture risk [34].

2.5 Garvan scale

Garvan scale (www.garvan.org.au) was devised to predict the absolute risk of OVCFs in 5 or 10 years in a given patient [35]. This tool does include age, sex, fractures after the age of 50, history of falls in the previous year, femoral neck BMD or T-score and weight. It differs from FRAX by including a history of falls and the number of previous fragility fractures. In addition to falls, multiple risk factors of OVCFs, including cardiovascular disease, type 2 diabetes, asthma, tricyclic antidepressants' usage and history of falls or liver disease, may make QFracture more advantageous in predicting individuals with internal medicine diseases.

2.6 Computed tomography (CT)

The risk assessment methods for OVCFs mentioned above remain underutilized. Computed tomography (CT) has been used to identify undiagnosed spinal osteoporosis in patients with lumbar degenerative diseases [36, 37]. The trabecular BMD assessed by CT provides a rapid and effective opportunistic screen for detecting individuals at increased risk for fragility fractures [38].

Recently, routine abdomen or chest CT scans were used for automatically assessing the feasibility of OVCFs risk [39]. Compared with FRAX for 5-year fracture risk, the CT-based predictor of major osteoporotic fracture presented better receiver operating characteristic area under curve (ROC AUC), sensitivity and positive predictive value.

In a word, the main task of risk assessment tools is to identify the individuals with a fracture risk high enough to justify anti-OP treatment, especially for those who did not yet suffer from a fracture and by administering anti-OP treatment to prevent OVCFs [40]. However, no optimal risk assessment tool available quantificationally identifies the OVCFs risk. More precise evaluation tools are needed to develop and quantitatively evaluate and predict the OVCFs risks in the future.

3. Primary drug treatment

3.1 Vitamin D

Vitamin D is essential for bone health and the functioning of systems of the human body. Vitamin D sufficiency refers to the serum concentration of vitamin D from 30 to 50 ng/ml (nanograms per milliliter) [41–43]. Endocrine Society suggested administering a daily vitamin D dose of 1500–2000 IU (international units), to reach the desired value of 30 ng/ml [44]. The association between serum concentration of vitamin D and bone health is described as follows: vitamin D deficiency (<25 nmol/L (nanomole per liter) produces a mineralization defect; vitamin D insufficiency (<50 nmol/L) produces secondary hyperparathyroidism and an increase in bone turnover [45–47]. Individuals who do not achieve the recommended dietary intake of calcium or vitamin D, especially those taking anti-OP medication, are advised to take supplements.

There is no single, fixed dose for all subjects to supplement. Most studies have investigated the efficacy of calcium and vitamin D on fracture risk but with inconsistent outcomes. Correcting vitamin D deficiencies and a serum concentration of 25-hydroxyvitamin D > 50 nmol/L can be beneficial [48]. However, there are little or no benefits in the supplements in individuals with sufficient vitamin D. A single oral high dose of vitamin D (such as 500,000 IU in autumn or winter annually) for 3 to 5 years was related to an increased risk of falls and fractures [49]. Except for malabsorption, the recommended dose should not exceed 4000 IU/day [49–51]. According to the Italian Society for Osteoporosis, Mineral Metabolism and Bone Diseases, the use of an initial loading dose (3000–10,000 IU/day, average 5000 IU/day for 1–2 months) was followed by the maintenance dose (2000 IU/day) in patients with serum 25(OH)D < 10 ng/ml, or in patients starting anti-OP therapy with intravenous bisphosphonates or denosumab with serum 25(OH)D < 20 ng/ml.

3.2 Calcium

Calcium is the main constituent of bone. Recommend a diet with adequate total calcium intake (1000 mg/day for men aged 50–70 years; 1200 mg/day for women ≥51 years and men≥71 years), incorporating calcium supplements if intake is insufficient [52]. Excessive intake of calcium (>1500 mg/day) might be associated with an increased risk of renal stones and cardiovascular events [53]. Calcium intake should be recommended in combination with vitamin D, and calcium supplementation alone does not affect increased BMD or decreased fracture risk [54].

4. Anti-OP therapy

4.1 Background

Either anti-resorptive or anabolic treatment is recommended by the US Food and Drug Administration for high-risk patients without contraindications following a risk assessment. Adequate intake of vitamin D and calcium is required in the anti-OP treatment. Both bisphosphonates (bone remodeling inhibitor) and denosumab (receptor activator of nuclear factor kappa-B ligand (RANKL inhibitor) are anti-resorptive agents to reduce the risk of hip, nonvertebral and vertebral fractures. Anabolic drugs, teriparatide and abaloparatide, are given by daily subcutaneous injection to stimulate bone formation. OVCFs risk is usually reduced by 30–70% following anti-OP treatment [26]. The benefit-to-risk ratio for anti-OP therapy is strongly positive for patients with osteoporosis.

4.2 Anti-resorptive therapies

4.2.1 Bisphosphonates

Bisphosphonates, the most used anti-OP drugs, reduce fracture risk by inhibiting bone remodeling. Generally, it is the first-line anti-OP agent in osteoporosis patients without contraindications. The progressively increased BMD has reached a plateau following 3–4 years of treatment [55, 56]. Other than zoledronic acid, the efficacy of anti-resorptive agents on the increased BMD is similar in both men and women. The benefits of decreasing fracture risks are retained after discontinuing alendronate or zoledronic acid. After 5 years of alendronate therapy and 3 years of zoledronic acid therapy, drug holidays are considered in patients with lower OVCFs risk [27]. Zoledronic acid treatment every 18 months for 6 years could effectively reduce the OVCFs risk [57]. A small note on bisphosphonate use should be limited to patients with a creatinine clearance >35 ml/min and serum vitamin D levels of 30–50 nmol/L to prevent symptomatic hypocalcemia [27, 58, 59]. Such adverse events as jaw osteonecrosis and atypical femoral fractures are related to bisphosphonates.

4.2.2 RANK ligand inhibitor

Denosumab, an osteocyte-derived regulator of osteoclast development binding to and inhibiting RANK ligand, reduces osteoclast activity to inhibit bone remodeling [60]. In postmenopausal women and men, a single dosage of 60 mg half-yearly administered by subcutaneous injection could effectively prevent the fracture risk of vertebrae, nonvertebrae and hip. The mineralization degree reaches a maximum by year 5 of treatment but by 10 years of treatment it results in greater BMD gains for sustainably protecting the vertebrae from fracture [61]. However, the BMD returns to baseline 18 months after the last injection [62, 63]. Treatment adherence is vital to maintaining the BMD, and note that alendronate or zoledronic acid administration is recommended for maintaining the efficacy of the prevention of OVCFs if denosumab treatment is discontinued [64, 65]. Rapid decreases in BMD were related to the loss of vertebral fracture protection, and multiple vertebral fractures have been reported to occur 3–18 months after stopping denosumab treatment [65].

Denosumab offers an alternative approach to the treatment of osteoporosis by decreasing bone resorption and increasing BMD through the inhibition of RANKL. Compared to bisphosphate, denosumab showed a stronger effect on inhibiting bone resorption and increasing BMD [66]. Denosumab rapidly inhibits bone resorption markers, which leads to an early and rapid decrease (within 24 h of treatment) in C-terminal telopeptide of type I collagen (CTX), followed by a later and smaller decrease in bone formation markers such as the N-terminal propeptide of type I procollagen (PINP) [67]. A reduction of CTX by 70–85% and PINP by 60–70% was found with anti-resorptive therapy [68, 69]. PINP and CTX were continuously suppressed with continuous administration for up to 8 years with a greater extent of PINP than CTX [70]. Compared with placebo, denosumab reduced the risk of vertebral fracture by 68%, hip fracture by 40% and nonvertebral fracture by 20% [71]. No serious adverse reaction, including cancer, infection, cardiovascular disease, fracture nonunion, hypocalcemia or jaw osteonecrosis, was found during the treatment period.

4.2.3 Hormone replacement therapy

The aim of estrogen treatment, with or without progestin, is to increase the BMD to reduce fracture risk at the hip, vertebrae and other sites in postmenopausal women [72]. The Women's Health Initiative randomized controlled trial indicated that the combined estrogen plus progestin could reduce the OVCFs by 34% [73]. A decreased use of estrogen is attributed to a balance of benefits and overall health risks between the efficacy of anti-OP and such extraskeletal effects as breast, endometrial, colorectal cancers, coronary heart disease, stroke and deep vein thrombosis. Guidelines recommend that the benefit-to-risk ratio is most favorable in women with elevated risk for bone loss or fracture in the age younger than 60 years or those who are within 10 years of menopause onset [74]. Treatment should be individualized using the best available evidence to maximize benefits and minimize risks, and it is advised to periodically reevaluate both the benefits and risks of continuing or discontinuing hormone replacement therapy.

4.2.4 Anabolic medications

Compared to anti-resorptive drugs, the anabolic agents of teriparatide and abaloparatide exert larger increases in vertebral BMD and have a stronger clinical efficacy in reducing OVCFs risk [75].

Teriparatide, a human parathyroid hormone (1–34), is used in patients with severe osteoporosis or complication to reduce the risk of new OVCFs by 65% [76]. It is advised to give the patient daily administration of teriparatide 20 μg by subcutaneous injection, and the longest medication duration time was 24 months because of the concerns of osteosarcoma. However, the US Food and Drug Administration now permits teriparatide use >2 years in patients at continuing high fracture risk, based on a study without increasing adult osteosarcoma incidence in a 15-Year US Postmarketing Surveillance Study [75, 77]. Increased spinal BMD with little effect on proximal femoral and distal radius BMD is the most striking feature (about 7%) following 2 years of treatment [78, 79]. In clinical trials in women with osteoporosis following teriparatide treatment for 21 months, vertebral and nonvertebral fractures were, respectively, reduced by two-thirds and one third, but with no significant reduction in hip fractures. In glucocorticoid-induced osteoporosis, it produces larger BMD increases than alendronate and substantially reduces vertebral, but not nonvertebral, fracture risk [80]. Upon discontinuing teriparatide therapy, an anti-resorptive agent, such as bisphosphonate or denosumab, is recommended to preserve the progressive increases in BMD [81]. PINP was a biological response marker during teriparatide treatment for osteoporosis and was used to assess treatment response [82, 83]. The changes in PINP are apparent as early as 3 days following the start of treatment [84]. A 30–50% increase in PINP with anabolic therapy is observed within months [85]. PINP levels increased following the teriparatide treatment and can be a surrogate marker of bone formation and strength [85]. PINP returned to around or below baseline levels by 28 days after stopping treatment [84]. A PINP value on treatment that is low (<35 μg/L) for anti-resorptive treatment or above 69 μg/L for anabolic therapy may be presumed to indicate adequate response [67].

Abaloparatide, available in the USA and Japan, is a selective activator of the Parathyroid Hormone 1 Receptor (PTH1R) and has a similar mechanism of action to teriparatide. Similar to teriparatide, abaloparatide is administered 80 μg daily by subcutaneous injection for up to 24 months.

4.2.5 Anti-sclerostin antibody therapies

Sclerostin, an osteocyte protein released at the bone surface, stimulates bone formation and inhibits bone resorption by inhibiting the wingless-type (Wnt) signaling in osteoblasts. The anabolic effect is achieved by an early and transient bone formation increase and a sustained bone resorption decrease [86].

Romosozumab, an anti-sclerostin monoclonal antibody, stimulates bone formation and inhibits resorption to increase BMD [86]. Subcutaneous injections of 210 mg/month for 12-month increase the BMD by 11.3% at the lumbar spine, compared to 7.1% with teriparatide (20 μg daily) and 4.1% with alendronate (70 mg weekly) [86]. Treatment for 12 months reduced the risk of vertebral and clinical fractures in postmenopausal osteoporosis women compared to a placebo [87]. And sequential treatment with denosumab further decreased the spinal fracture risk, providing a foundation for an ongoing reduction in the OVCFs risk during sequential treatment with denosumab. As to the risk of hip fractures, romosozumab followed by alendronate treatment resulted in a significantly lower risk than alendronate alone, suggesting an important benefit and challenging the common treatment practice of first-line use of alendronate [88].

5. Monitoring anti-OP treatment

5.1 Background

Anti-OP treatment aims to improve the BMD to reduce OVCFs risk. Prevention of fracture is the predominant outcome following anti-OP treatment. Hence, monitoring anti-OP treatment is vital for successful osteoporosis management. The changes in BMD are affected by bone turnover. Bone turnover is comprised of two processes including bone resorption and bone formation. The decreased bone resorption or/and increased bone formation could affect the changes in BMD. Bone turnover markers

(BTMs) are used to assess the changes in bone resorption and formation. Fractures are the gold standard for measuring efficacy and changes in BMD, and BTMs could be served as surrogates [89]. Hence, the assessment of changes in bone turnover as well as BMD was used to monitor anti-OP treatment.

In an attempt to better monitor the efficacy of anti-OP treatment, requirements for anti-OP treatment are listed below [89]:

1. Anti-OP therapy was well tolerated.
2. Intake of adequate calcium and vitamin D.
3. A treatment period of at least 1 year to become fully effective.

5.2 BMD

Osteoporosis is characterized by progressive loss of bone, and BMD is a predictor of fracture risk. There is a strong, continuous relationship between the BMD and OVCFs, the greater the increased BMD, the lower the fracture risk [90, 91]. Early monitoring of anti-OP treatment efficacy is very important to guide anti-OP treatment. However, the changes in BMD are difficult to detect at an early treatment stage. According to the clinical circumstances, BMD testing is commonly performed 1 year after the anti-OP therapy and at appropriate intervals thereafter.

Based on the changes in BMD and new fracture, treatment response was clarified as three categories [89]: inadequate response (incident fracture and a decrease in BMD greater than 2%), possible inadequate response (incident fracture and a decrease in BMD greater than 2%) and adequate response (no fracture and no decrease in BMD greater than 2%). The Committee of Scientific Advisors of International Osteoporosis Foundation (IOF) recommended that the treatment should be changed to 4% decline in BMD at the lumbar spine after at least two serial BMD measurements [92].

5.3 BTMs

Anti-OP agents exert their effect by influencing the bone formation and/or bone resorption. The International Osteoporosis Foundation (IOF) and the International Federation of Clinical Chemistry (IFCC) have recommended serum PINP and CTX as reference bone turnover markers. Bone turnover markers hold promise in fracture risk prediction and monitoring treatment [93, 94]. The use of BTMs for the monitoring of treatment requires a baseline assessment with a repeat measurement at some defined point during treatment. In people with osteoporosis, bone turnover markers might be useful to assess the response to anabolic and anti-resorptive therapies, assess compliance to therapy or indicate possible secondary osteoporosis. Several studies have described the relationship between the reduction in bone turnover markers following anti-resorptive therapy and the reduction in vertebral and nonvertebral fracture risk [95, 96]. Increased concentrations of bone turnover markers can be associated with increased rates of bone loss and fracture risk [93]. In patients receiving teriparatide treatment, the changes in serum levels of PINP were significantly correlated with vertebral bone strength, which indicates that serum PINP monitoring could serve as a surrogate marker of biomechanical properties in clinical practice [85].

The Committee of Scientific Advisors of IOF recommended that a significant response is a decline of 25% from baseline levels for anti-resorptive treatments and a 25% increase for anabolic agents after 6 months [92]. For anti-resorptive treatments, if baseline levels are not known, a positive response is a decrease below the average value of young healthy adults. It is assumed that the response is similar between men and women [92].

5.4 CT

The CT Hounsfield unit values of the vertebra have been used for the assessment of vertebral BMD [38]. In the previous studies, the vertebral CT values increase significantly following anti-OP treatment [17]. Here, we suggest that vertebral CT values could be used as a method for monitoring anti-OP treatment.

6. OVCFs therapy

6.1 Treatment goal

The primary treatment goal is to improve spinal BMD to boost fracture union, prevent vertebral collapse, relieve back pain and prevent new OVCFs. Improving the HRQoL is the ultimate aim following OVCFs.

6.2 Conservative treatment

Traditional conservative treatment, including brace treatment and pain relief, is an option for symptomatic OVCFs [97]. Bracing is the standard conservative treatment for acute OVCFs to immobilize the fracture site to manage pain and boost the OVCFs healing, resulting in the least residual pain and disability in the long term [98]. Routine use of a custom-made rigid brace for acute OVCFs is not recommended [99]. For acute OVCFs patients, rigid-brace treatment did not result in better prevention of spinal kyphotic deformities, better HRQoL or lesser back pain than soft brace. Bed rest was not recommended during OVCFs treatment [52].

However, approximately 30–40% of patients still experience severe low back pain [100, 101]. Calcitonin salmon has been shown to dramatically reduce acute pain due to acute OVCFs. Recent studies indicate that the paravertebral muscles play a substantial role in back pain, sagittal balance and HRQoL [102]. Low back pain at the 6-month follow-up was higher in patients with paravertebral muscle decline. Once the acute pain improves, patients are recommended to exercise paravertebral muscles for chronic back pain.

Conservative treatment for OVCF carries inherent risks. Treatment failure was not rare in clinical practice, such as the progression of collapse, kyphotic deformity, fracture nonunion and neurologic impairment. BMD T value less than −3.45 and the presence of intravertebral cleft were high-risk factors for conservative treatment failure [103]. In addition, the shape of the OVCFs vertebrae, the middle column damage and the involvement of thoracolumbar junction can also be predictors for vertebral collapse and nonunion of OVCFs [104]. A diffuse low-type pattern on T1-weighted MRI and diffuse low- and fluid-type patterns on T2-weighted MRI were independent risk factors for nonunion of acute OVCFs [105]. Acute OVCFs with these risk factors should be actively observed for nonunion and vertebral collapse.

6.3 Surgery treatment

Vertebral augmentation procedures (VAPs) were recommended for patients with severe back pain or no response to conservative treatment [106]. Being the immediate postoperative pain relief, VAP was widely applied to restore intravertebral stability following the injection of bone cement into the fractured vertebrae and recommended by the Cardiovascular and Interventional Radiological Society of Europe for OVCF treatment [107]. Detailed surgical techniques will not be presented in this section. Based on a meta-analysis, the clinical efficacy showed that OVCFs patients who underwent VAP treatment were 22% less likely to die at up to 10 years than those receiving nonsurgical treatment [106]. However, the prevalence of severe complications related to VAP could be as high as 12.5–36.8% [108–112]. The most common complications encountered are cement leakage and new OVCFs at the adjacent level. Higher viscosity and less cement were recommended to reduce the leakage risk and related complications [113]. New OVCFs of cemented vertebrae after VAP were about 63%, and the greater the anterior vertebral height obtained, the greater the risk of refracture occurring [18]. Other cement-related complications, including pulmonary embolism, spinal cord burn, adjacent vertebrae collapse and cement migration, were not rare [110, 114, 115]. Besides, patients who received VAP should be informed about the clinical effect and the subsequent anti-OP treatment was also administered to reduce the risk of new OVCFs [116].

However, VAP remains a controversial treatment. Although extensively used for OVCFs, VAP was not recommended based on recent studies [116, 117]. Compared with placebo control, the efficacy of VAP in pain control was less than 6 weeks [118]. Recent high- to moderate-quality evidence indicates that VAP does not offer significant clinical benefits compared with the sham procedure [117, 119, 120]. One challenge was that VAP treatment only targeted the restoration of stability of the fractured vertebrae and did not improve spinal BMD to decrease the fracture risk of the treated or nontreated vertebrae [18]. Another challenge is that VAP is not suitable for patients with surgical contraindications [121]. The anti-osteoporotic treatment administered following VAP could reduce the risk of refracture by 40–70% [116].

Obviously, VAP was not suitable for OVCFs. The goal of OVCFs treatment is to relieve back pain, boost OVCFs union, improve spinal BMD to decrease the risk of refracture and improve the HRQoL. In addition, the fracture healing vertebrae significantly related to relieved back pain, compared to the patients without bone union [122].

Now that anti-OP therapy is still needed after VAP, selecting an anti-OP therapy method that can promote bone healing as well as prevent refracture is a better treatment. Thus, obtaining similar therapeutic effects to VAP with lesser complication and cost, no matter patients with or without surgical contraindications [123].

6.4 Teriparatide treatment

As far as the clinical efficacy of anti-OP treatment is concerned, the clinical benefits of teriparatide treatment had been confirmed by stimulating new bone formation to increase BMD and strength to prevent OVCFs [76]. Bisphosphonate use does not significantly affect the clinical results during conservative treatment for OVCFs, as well as the occurrence of the nonunion was related to medication history [124]. So, we do not recommend bisphosphonate use during the fracture union period. Recently, teriparatide treatment gradually showed its clinical advantage on

OVCFs in clinical practice [125, 126]. In patients with neurological deficits following new unstable OVCF and surgical contraindications, teriparatide treatment was better than alendronate at improving the BMD and preventing aggravation of spinal cord compromise [121]. In postmenopausal women with OVCFs, teriparatide treatment was related to the consequent back pain alleviation and improved HRQoL [1]. The signal changes in bone marrow following treatment on magnetic resonance imaging (MRI) could reflect the role of enhancing fracture healing at 3 months posttreatment.

The Union of OVCFs following teriparatide treatment was first quantitatively assessed with CT images in our previous study [17, 127, 128]. Teriparatide treatment for OVCFs proved effective in remission of back pain by boosting fracture union, prevention of progressive vertebral collapse and new OVCFs and improvement in the HRQoL [17]. At least 1 year of treatment indicated that the clinical effect on back pain, spinal function, BMD and new OVCFs was superior to that of VAP, but with no requirements for hospitalization [17]. A typical acute OVCF case following teriparatide treatment is shown in **Figure 1**.

7. Nonunion of OVCFs therapy

7.1 Background

Like other fractures, OVCFs may develop nonunion with an incidence of 10–48% [129–131]. The fracture nonunion was defined as an intravertebral vacuum cleft detected within a deformed vertebral body at least 4 months after the fracture event, in which the signals displayed hypointensity on T1- and T2-weighted and fat-suppressed sequences [127, 132–134]. Once nonunion occurs, patients may suffer from intractable back pain and neurological deficits caused by intravertebral instability, leading to a further reduced HRQoL and increased mortality [23, 24].

Although the nonunion of OVCFs is called by most scholars as Kümmell's disease, research showed that they are two different diseases now [135–137]. The main cornerstones of Kümmell's disease must be a history of trauma with a negative spinal

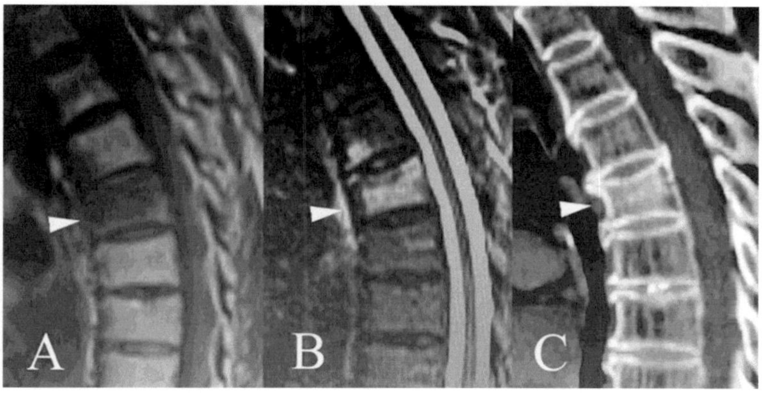

Figure 1.
Teriparatide treatment boosts T7 OVCF union in a 70-year-old female patient. The hypointensity on sagittal T1-weighted (A, white arrow) and hyperintensity on fat-suppressed sequence (B, white arrow) within the T7 show acute OVCF. Sagittal CT image of T7 vertebral body (C, white arrow) at month 4 following teriparatide treatment shows intravertebral bone formation connecting the upper and lower endplates, indicating the fracture union.

radiological investigation, an asymptomatic period followed by the intravertebral vacuum cleft [138]. Based on our research, the initial factor for Kümmell's disease was not undisplaced OVCFs but a magnetic resonance imaging of negative spine trauma that progressed into a delayed vertebral collapse with intravertebral vacuum cleft [128].

7.2 Treatment goal

The treatment goal of fracture nonunion treatment is to restore intravertebral stability by cement technique, vertebral body replacement, long- or short-level screw fixation or the promotion of fracture union. The OVCFs nonunion was often refractory to conservative treatment. So far, no standard or single treatment is yet available.

7.3 Surgery treatment

Open operation or VAP was recommended in patients with no response to conservative treatment, including severe back pain, worsening neurological deficits or progressive spinal kyphosis [106].

Traditional open internal fixation, including a posterior, anterior and a combined approach, was used to relieve the clinical symptoms. However, severe osteoporosis often accompanies this fracture nonunion in these aged patients, and medical complications may also be present. The osteoporotic vertebrae could not hold the implanted pedicle screws and titanium cage, leading to internal fixation or intervertebral fusion failure.

Less invasive VAP was widely applied for OVCFs nonunion, recommended by the Cardiovascular and Interventional Radiological Society of Europe for OVCF treatment [107]. VAP could relieve back pain, restore vertebral height and correct spinal kyphosis to an extent. However, patients with nerve damage from spinal canal stenosis were likely not to benefit from invasive treatment, with the risk of cement leakage and neurological damage.

Some studies have found that patients may not benefit from VAP. VAP for nonunion of OVCFs, the same as OVCFs, remains a controversial treatment. In addition, more complications are another challenge. Like OVCFs, anti-OP is still needed after VP.

7.4 Teriparatide treatment

The main clinical symptom, including persistent pain and spinal cord deficits, is intravertebral instability from the nonunion [129, 139, 140]. We believe that restoration of the intravertebral stability by enhancing the fracture union may be more suitable for the nonunion of OVCFs. Assessment of fracture union following teriparatide treatment for at least 6 months was quantified on sagittal CT images in our previous study [127]. Our research indicated that teriparatide treatment could boot fracture union and prevent progressive vertebral collapse [127, 132]. All the clinical symptoms were relieved following the fracture union. Besides, the increased spinal BMD to prevent new OVCFs and improve the HRQoL was also observed in the study. At least 6 months of teriparatide treatment may be a choice for the nonunion of OVCF.

8. Conclusions

Osteoporosis is a chronic and long-term condition that even requires lifelong management. The anti-OP management to prevent OVCFs is one of the most important objectives. The fracture risk assessment tools were used to assess the fracture risk and direct subsequent anti-OP therapy. In elderly populations with a high risk of fracture, early anti-OP with bisphosphonates or denosumab is efficient in decreasing the OVCFs risk. Teriparatide or abaloparatide treatment followed by anti-resorptive agent treatment may be more suitable for those with high or imminent fracture risk. Although VAP is extensively used either in OVCFs or nonunion patients, anabolic medications gradually showed clinical efficacy in enhancing fracture union. Despite substantial advances in treatment options to reduce OVCF risk, many high-risk individuals have not given enough attention. Offering individualized, efficient and safe treatment regimens remains a challenge for the future.

Funding

The Basic Research Program of Shanxi Province, China (grants 202203021221264) supported this research.

Conflict of interest

The authors declare no conflict of interest.

Author details

Pengguo Gou* and Feng Chang*
Department of Orthopaedic Surgery, The Fifth Hospital of Shanxi Medical University, Taiyuan, Shanxi, China

*Address all correspondence to: 763146351@qq.com and cfmedmail@163.com

References

[1] Chen Z, Lin W, Zhao S, Mo X, Yuan W, Cheung WH, et al. Effect of teriparatide on pain relief, and quality of life in postmenopausal females with osteoporotic vertebral compression fractures, a retrospective cohort study. Annals of Palliative Medicine. 2021;**10**:4000-4007. DOI: 10.21037/apm-20-2333

[2] Ruiz-Adame M, Correa M. A systematic review of the indirect and social costs studies in fragility fractures. Osteoporosis International. 2020;**31**:1205-1216. DOI: 10.1007/s00198-020-05319-x

[3] Ballane G, Cauley JA, Luckey MM, El-Hajj FG. Worldwide prevalence and incidence of osteoporotic vertebral fractures. Osteoporosis International. 2017;**28**:1531-1542. DOI: 10.1007/s00198-017-3909-3

[4] Hoffmann DB, Popescu C, Komrakova M, Welte L, Saul D, Lehmann W, et al. Chronic hyponatremia in patients with proximal femoral fractures after low energy trauma: A retrospective study in a level-1 trauma center. Bone Report. 2020;**12**:100234. DOI: 10.1016/j.bonr.2019.100234

[5] Kim SM, Yeom JW, Song HK, Hwang KT, Hwang JH, Yoo JH. Lateral locked plating for distal femur fractures by low-energy trauma: What makes a difference in healing? International Orthopaedics. 2018;**42**:2907-2914. DOI: 10.1007/s00264-018-3881-3

[6] Genant HK, Cooper C, Poor G, et al. Interim report and recommendations of the World Health Organization task-force for osteoporosis. Osteoporosis International. 1999;**10**:259-264. DOI: 10.1007/s001980050224

[7] Karmakar A, Acharya S, Biswas D, Sau A. Evaluation of percutaneous vertebroplasty for management of symptomatic osteoporotic compression fracture. Journal of Clinical and Diagnostic Research. 2017;**11**:RC07-RC10. DOI: 10.7860/JCDR/2017/25886.10461

[8] Schousboe JT. Epidemiology of vertebral fractures. Journal of Clinical Densitometry. 2016;**19**:8-22. DOI: 10.1016/j.jocd.2015.08.004

[9] Zeytinoglu M, Jain RK, Vokes TJ. Vertebral fracture assessment: Enhancing the diagnosis, prevention, and treatment of osteoporosis. Bone. 2017;**104**:54-65. DOI: 10.1016/j.bone.2017.03.004

[10] Borgstrom F, Olafsson G, Strom O, Tillman JB, Wardlaw D, Boonen S, et al. The impact of different health dimensions on overall quality of life related to kyphoplasty and non-surgical management. Osteoporosis International. 2013;**24**:1991-1999. DOI: 10.1007/s00198-012-2237-x

[11] Si L, Winzenberg TM, de Graaff B, Palmer AJ. A systematic review and meta-analysis of utility-based quality of life for osteoporosis-related conditions. Osteoporosis International. 2014;**25**:1987-1997. DOI: 10.1007/s00198-014-2636-2

[12] Ross PD, Ettinger B, Davis JW, Melton LJ 3rd, Wasnich RD. Evaluation of adverse health outcomes associated with vertebral fractures. Osteoporosis International. 1991;**1**:134-140. DOI: 10.1007/BF01625442

[13] Mauch JT, Carr CM, Cloft H, Diehn FE. Review of the imaging features of benign osteoporotic and malignant vertebral compression fractures. AJNR.

American Journal of Neuroradiology. 2018;**39**:1584-1592. DOI: 10.3174/ajnr.A5528

[14] Takahashi S, Hoshino M, Takayama K, et al. Predicting delayed union in osteoporotic vertebral fractures with consecutive magnetic resonance imaging in the acute phase: A multicenter cohort study. Osteoporosis International. 2016;**27**:3567-3575. DOI: 10.1007/s00198-016-3687-3

[15] Marongiu G, Congia S, Verona M, Lombardo M, Podda D, Capone A. The impact of magnetic resonance imaging in the diagnostic and classification process of osteoporotic vertebral fractures. Injury. 2018;**49**(Suppl. 3):S26-S31. DOI: 10.1016/j.injury.2018.10.006

[16] Miller PD. Management of severe osteoporosis. Expert Opinion on Pharmacotherapy. 2016;**17**:473-488. DOI: 10.1517/14656566.2016.1124856

[17] Gou P, Zhao Z, Yu C, Hou X, Gao G, Zhang T, et al. Efficacy of recombinant human parathyroid hormone versus vertebral augmentation procedure on patients with acute osteoporotic vertebral compression fracture. Orthopaedic Surgery. 2022;**14**:2510-2518. DOI: 10.1111/os.13470

[18] Lin WC, Lee YC, Lee CH, Kuo YL, Cheng YF, Lui CC, et al. Refractures in cemented vertebrae after percutaneous vertebroplasty: A retrospective analysis. European Spine Journal. 2008;**17**:592-599. DOI: 10.1007/s00586-007-0564-y

[19] Lavelle WF, Cheney R. Recurrent fracture after vertebral kyphoplasty. The Spine Journal. 2006;**6**:488-493. DOI: 10.1016/j.spinee.2005.10.013

[20] Lunt M, O'Neill TW, Felsenberg D, Reeve J, Kanis JA, Cooper C, et al. Characteristics of a prevalent vertebral deformity predict subsequent vertebral fracture: Results from the European Prospective Osteoporosis Study (EPOS). Bone. 2003;**33**:505-513. DOI: 10.1016/s8756-3282(03)00248-5

[21] Lindsay R, Silverman SL, Cooper C, et al. Risk of new vertebral fracture in the year following a fracture. Journal of the American Medical Association. 2001;**285**:320-323. DOI: 10.1001/jama.285.3.320

[22] Wong CC, McGirt MJ. Vertebral compression fractures: A review of current management and multimodal therapy. Journal of Multidisciplinary Healthcare. 2013;**6**:205-214. DOI: 10.2147/JMDH.S31659

[23] Edidin AA, Ong KL, Lau E, Kurtz SM. Morbidity and mortality after vertebral fractures: Comparison of vertebral augmentation and nonoperative management in the medicare population. Spine (Phila Pa 1976). 2015;**40**:1228-1241. DOI: 10.1097/BRS.0000000000000992

[24] Lim J, Choi SW, Youm JY, Kwon HJ, Kim SH, Koh HS. Posttraumatic delayed vertebral collapse: Kummell's disease. Journal of Korean Neurosurgical Association. 2018;**61**:1-9. DOI: 10.3340/jkns.2017.0505.010

[25] Bliuc D, Nguyen ND, Milch VE, Nguyen TV, Eisman JA, Center JR. Mortality risk associated with low-trauma osteoporotic fracture and subsequent fracture in men and women. Journal of the American Medical Association. 2009;**301**:513-521. DOI: 10.1001/jama.2009.50

[26] Compston JE, McClung MR, Leslie WD. Osteoporosis. Lancet. 2019;**393**:364-376. DOI: 10.1016/S0140-6736(18)32112-3

[27] Black DM, Rosen CJ. Clinical practice: Postmenopausal osteoporosis. New England Journal of Medicine. 2016;**374**:254-262. DOI: 10.1056/NEJMcp1513724

[28] van Geel TA, van Helden S, Geusens PP, Winkens B, Dinant GJ. Clinical subsequent fractures cluster in time after first fractures. Annals of the Rheumatic Diseases. 2009;**68**:99-102. DOI: 10.1136/ard.2008.092775

[29] Siris ES, Chen YT, Abbott TA, Barrett-Connor E, Miller PD, Wehren LE, et al. Bone mineral density thresholds for pharmacological intervention to prevent fractures. Archives of Internal Medicine. 2004;**164**:1108-1112. DOI: 10.1001/archinte.164.10.1108

[30] Schuit SC, van der Klift M, Weel AE, de Laet CE, Burger H, Seeman E, et al. Fracture incidence and association with bone mineral density in elderly men and women: The Rotterdam study. Bone. 2004;**34**:195-202. DOI: 10.1016/j.bone.2003.10.001

[31] Kanis JA, Johnell O, Oden A, Johansson H, McCloskey E. FRAX and the assessment of fracture probability in men and women from the UK. Osteoporosis International. 2008;**19**:385-397. DOI: 10.1007/s00198-007-0543-5

[32] Middleton RG, Shabani F, Uzoigwe CE, Shoaib A, Moqsith M, Venkatesan M. FRAX and the assessment of the risk of developing a fragility fracture. Journal of Bone and Joint Surgery. British Volume (London). 2012;**94**:1313-1320. DOI: 10.1302/0301-620X.94B10.28889

[33] Kanis JA, Hans D, Cooper C, et al. Interpretation and use of FRAX in clinical practice. Osteoporosis International. 2011;**22**:2395-2411. DOI: 10.1007/s00198-011-1713-z

[34] Kanis JA, Harvey NC, Johansson H, Oden A, McCloskey EV, Leslie WD. Overview of fracture prediction tools. Journal of Clinical Densitometry. 2017;**20**:444-450. DOI: 10.1016/j.jocd.2017.06.013

[35] Crandall CJ. Risk assessment tools for osteoporosis screening in postmenopausal women: A systematic review. Current Osteoporosis Reports. 2015;**13**:287-301. DOI: 10.1007/s11914-015-0282-z

[36] Engelke K, Chaudry O, Bartenschlager S. Opportunistic screening techniques for analysis of CT scans. Current Osteoporosis Reports. 2023;**21**:65-76. DOI: 10.1007/s11914-022-00764-5

[37] Zou D, Li W, Deng C, Du G, Xu N. The use of CT Hounsfield unit values to identify the undiagnosed spinal osteoporosis in patients with lumbar degenerative diseases. European Spine Journal. 2019;**28**:1758-1766. DOI: 10.1007/s00586-018-5776-9

[38] Lee S, Binkley N, Lubner M, Bruce R, Ziemlewicz T, Pickhardt P. Opportunistic screening for osteoporosis using the sagittal reconstruction from routine abdominal CT for combined assessment of vertebral fractures and density. Osteoporosis International. 2016;**27**:1131-1136. DOI: 10.1007/s00198-015-3318-4

[39] Dagan N, Elnekave E, Barda N, Bregman-Amitai O, Bar A, Orlovsky M, et al. Automated opportunistic osteoporotic fracture risk assessment using computed tomography scans to aid in FRAX underutilization. Nature Medicine. 2020;**26**:77-82. DOI: 10.1038/s41591-019-0720-z

[40] Cozadd AJ, Schroder LK, Switzer JA. Fracture risk assessment: An update. The Journal of Bone and Joint Surgery.

American Volume. 2021;**103**:1238-1246. DOI: 10.2106/JBJS.20.01071

[41] Holick MF, Binkley NC, Bischoff-Ferrari HA, Gordon CM, Hanley DA, Heaney RP, et al. Evaluation, treatment, and prevention of vitamin D deficiency: An Endocrine Society clinical practice guideline. The Journal of Clinical Endocrinology and Metabolism. 2011;**96**:1911-1930. DOI: 10.1210/jc.2011-0385

[42] Dudenkov DV, Yawn BP, Oberhelman SS, Fischer PR, Singh RJ, Cha SS, et al. Changing incidence of serum 25-hydroxyvitamin D values above 50 ng/mL: A 10-year population-based study. Mayo Clinic Proceedings. 2015;**90**:577-586. DOI: 10.1016/j.mayocp.2015.02.012

[43] Bertoldo F, Cianferotti L, Di Monaco M, et al. Definition, assessment, and management of vitamin D inadequacy: Suggestions, recommendations, and warnings from the Italian Society for Osteoporosis, Mineral Metabolism and Bone Diseases (SIOMMMS). Nutrients. 2022;**14**:4148. DOI: 10.3390/nu14194148

[44] Holick MF, Binkley NC, Bischoff-Ferrari HA, Gordon CM, Hanley DA, Heaney RP, et al. Guidelines for preventing and treating vitamin D deficiency and insufficiency revisited. The Journal of Clinical Endocrinology and Metabolism. 2012;**97**:1153-1158. DOI: 10.1210/jc.2011-2601

[45] Cranney A, Horsley T, O'Donnell S, et al. Effectiveness and safety of vitamin D in relation to bone health. Evidence Report/Technology Assessment. 2007;(158):1-235

[46] Fernandez H, Mohammed HT, Patel T. Vitamin D supplementation for bone health in adults with epilepsy: A systematic review. Epilepsia. 2018;**59**:885-896. DOI: 10.1111/epi.14015

[47] Jean G, Souberbielle JC, Chazot C. Vitamin D in chronic kidney disease and dialysis patients. Nutrients. 2017;**9**:328. DOI: 10.3390/nu9040328

[48] Bouillon R. Safety of high-dose vitamin D supplementation. The Journal of Clinical Endocrinology and Metabolism. 2020;**105**:1290-1291. DOI: 10.1210/clinem/dgz282

[49] Sanders KM, Stuart AL, Williamson EJ, Simpson JA, Kotowicz MA, Young D, et al. Annual high-dose oral vitamin D and falls and fractures in older women: A randomized controlled trial. Journal of the American Medical Association. 2010;**303**:1815-1822. DOI: 10.1001/jama.2010.594

[50] Ross AC, Manson JE, Abrams SA, et al. The 2011 report on dietary reference intakes for calcium and vitamin D from the Institute of Medicine: What clinicians need to know. The Journal of Clinical Endocrinology and Metabolism. 2011;**96**:53-58. DOI: 10.1210/jc.2010-2704

[51] Bischoff-Ferrari HA, Dawson-Hughes B, Orav EJ, Staehelin HB, Meyer OW, Theiler R, et al. Monthly high-dose vitamin D treatment for the prevention of functional decline: A randomized clinical trial. JAMA Internal Medicine. 2016;**176**:175-183. DOI: 10.1001/jamainternmed.2015.7148

[52] LeBoff MS, Greenspan SL, Insogna KL, Lewiecki EM, Saag KG, Singer AJ, et al. The clinician's guide to prevention and treatment of osteoporosis. Osteoporosis International. 2022;**33**:2049-2102. DOI: 10.1007/s00198-021-05900-y

[53] Jackson RD, LaCroix AZ, Gass M, et al. Calcium plus vitamin D

supplementation and the risk of fractures. The New England Journal of Medicine. 2006;**354**:669-683. DOI: 10.1056/NEJMoa055218

[54] Bailey RL, Zou P, Wallace TC, McCabe GP, Craig BA, Jun S, et al. Calcium supplement use is associated with less bone mineral density loss, but does not lessen the risk of bone fracture across the menopause transition: Data from the study of women's health across the Nation. JBMR Plus. 2020;**4**:e10246. DOI: 10.1002/jbm4.10246

[55] Black DM, Schwartz AV, Ensrud KE, et al. Effects of continuing or stopping alendronate after 5 years of treatment: The fracture intervention trial long-term extension (FLEX): A randomized trial. Journal of the American Medical Association. 2006;**296**:2927-2938. DOI: 10.1001/jama.296.24.2927

[56] Black DM, Reid IR, Cauley JA, et al. The effect of 6 versus 9 years of zoledronic acid treatment in osteoporosis: A randomized second extension to the HORIZON-pivotal fracture trial (PFT). Journal of Bone and Mineral Research. 2015;**30**:934-944. DOI: 10.1002/jbmr.2442

[57] Reid IR, Horne AM, Mihov B, Stewart A, Garratt E, Wong S, et al. Fracture prevention with zoledronate in older women with osteopenia. The New England Journal of Medicine. 2018;**379**:2407-2416. DOI: 10.1056/NEJMoa1808082

[58] Robinson DE, Ali MS, Pallares N, et al. Safety of oral bisphosphonates in moderate-to-severe chronic kidney disease: A binational cohort analysis. Journal of Bone and Mineral Research. 2021;**36**:820-832. DOI: 10.1002/jbmr.4235

[59] Evenepoel P, Cunningham J, Ferrari S, et al. European consensus statement on the diagnosis and management of osteoporosis in chronic kidney disease stages G4-G5D. Nephrology, Dialysis, Transplantation. 2021;**36**:42-59. DOI: 10.1093/ndt/gfaa192

[60] Rachner TD, Khosla S, Hofbauer LC. Osteoporosis: Now and the future. Lancet. 2011;**377**:1276-1287. DOI: 10.1016/S0140-6736(10)62349-5

[61] Bone HG, Wagman RB, Brandi ML, et al. 10 years of denosumab treatment in postmenopausal women with osteoporosis: Results from the phase 3 randomised FREEDOM trial and open-label extension. The Lancet Diabetes and Endocrinology. 2017;**5**:513-523. DOI: 10.1016/S2213-8587(17)30138-9

[62] Popp AW, Varathan N, Buffat H, Senn C, Perrelet R, Lippuner K. Bone mineral density changes after 1 year of denosumab discontinuation in postmenopausal women with long-term denosumab treatment for osteoporosis. Calcified Tissue International. 2018;**103**:50-54. DOI: 10.1007/s00223-018-0394-4

[63] Bone HG, Bolognese MA, Yuen CK, Kendler DL, Miller PD, Yang YC, et al. Effects of denosumab treatment and discontinuation on bone mineral density and bone turnover markers in postmenopausal women with low bone mass. The Journal of Clinical Endocrinology and Metabolism. 2011;**96**:972-980. DOI: 10.1210/jc.2010-1502

[64] Tutaworn T, Nieves JW, Wang Z, Levin JE, Yoo JE, Lane JM. Bone loss after denosumab discontinuation is prevented by alendronate and zoledronic acid but not risedronate: A retrospective study. Osteoporosis International. 2023;**34**:573-584. DOI: 10.1007/s00198-022-06648-9

[65] Cummings SR, Ferrari S, Eastell R, et al. Vertebral fractures after

discontinuation of denosumab: A post hoc analysis of the randomized placebo-controlled FREEDOM trial and its extension. Journal of Bone and Mineral Research. 2018;**33**:190-198. DOI: 10.1002/jbmr.3337

[66] Miller PD, Pannacciulli N, Brown JP, et al. Denosumab or zoledronic acid in postmenopausal women with osteoporosis previously treated with oral bisphosphonates. The Journal of Clinical Endocrinology and Metabolism. 2016;**101**:3163-3170. DOI: 10.1210/jc.2016-1801

[67] Eastell R, Pigott T, Gossiel F, Naylor KE, Walsh JS, Peel NFA. Diagnosis of endocrine disease: Bone turnover markers: Are they clinically useful? European Journal of Endocrinology. 2018;**178**:R19-R31. DOI: 10.1530/EJE-17-0585

[68] Camacho PM, Lopez NA. Use of biochemical markers of bone turnover in the management of postmenopausal osteoporosis. Clinical Chemistry and Laboratory Medicine. 2008;**46**:1345-1357. DOI: 10.1515/CCLM.2008.310

[69] Szulc P, Naylor K, Hoyle NR, Eastell R, Leary ET, National Bone Health Alliance Bone Turnover Marker P. Use of CTX-I and PINP as bone turnover markers: National bone health alliance recommendations to standardize sample handling and patient preparation to reduce pre-analytical variability. Osteoporosis International. 2017;**28**:2541-2556. DOI: 10.1007/s00198-017-4082-4

[70] Papapoulos S, Lippuner K, Roux C, et al. The effect of 8 or 5 years of denosumab treatment in postmenopausal women with osteoporosis: Results from the FREEDOM extension study. Osteoporosis International. 2015;**26**:2773-2783. DOI: 10.1007/s00198-015-3234-7

[71] Cummings SR, San Martin J, McClung MR, et al. Denosumab for prevention of fractures in postmenopausal women with osteoporosis. The New England Journal of Medicine. 2009;**361**:756-765. DOI: 10.1056/NEJMoa0809493

[72] Cauley JA, Robbins J, Chen Z, et al. Effects of estrogen plus progestin on risk of fracture and bone mineral density: The women's health initiative randomized trial. Journal of the American Medical Association. 2003;**290**:1729-1738. DOI: 10.1001/jama.290.13.1729

[73] Rossouw JE, Anderson GL, Prentice RL, et al. Risks and benefits of estrogen plus progestin in healthy postmenopausal women: Principal results from the women's health initiative randomized controlled trial. Journal of the American Medical Association. 2002;**288**:321-333. DOI: 10.1001/jama.288.3.321

[74] The NHTPSAP. Hormone therapy position statement of the North American Menopause Society. Menopause. 2017;**24**:728-753. DOI: 10.1097/GME.0000000000000921

[75] Reid IR, Billington EO. Drug therapy for osteoporosis in older adults. Lancet. 2022;**399**:1080-1092. DOI: 10.1016/S0140-6736(21)02646-5

[76] Neer RM, Arnaud CD, Zanchetta JR, et al. Effect of parathyroid hormone (1-34) on fractures and bone mineral density in postmenopausal women with osteoporosis. The New England Journal of Medicine. 2001;**344**:1434-1441. DOI: 10.1056/NEJM200105103441904

[77] Gilsenan A, Midkiff K, Harris D, Kellier-Steele N, McSorley D, Andrews EB. Teriparatide did not increase adult osteosarcoma incidence in a 15-year US postmarketing

surveillance study. Journal of Bone and Mineral Research. 2021;**36**:244-251. DOI: 10.1002/jbmr.4188

[78] Langdahl BL, Libanati C, Crittenden DB, et al. Romosozumab (sclerostin monoclonal antibody) versus teriparatide in postmenopausal women with osteoporosis transitioning from oral bisphosphonate therapy: A randomised, open-label, phase 3 trial. Lancet. 2017;**390**:1585-1594. DOI: 10.1016/S0140-6736(17)31613-6

[79] Leder BZ, Tsai JN, Uihlein AV, Wallace PM, Lee H, Neer RM, et al. Denosumab and teriparatide transitions in postmenopausal osteoporosis (the DATA-switch study): Extension of a randomised controlled trial. Lancet. 2015;**386**:1147-1155. DOI: 10.1016/S0140-6736(15)61120-5

[80] Saag KG, Shane E, Boonen S, Marin F, Donley DW, Taylor KA, et al. Teriparatide or alendronate in glucocorticoid-induced osteoporosis. The New England Journal of Medicine. 2007;**357**:2028-2039. DOI: 10.1056/NEJMoa071408

[81] McClung MR. Using osteoporosis therapies in combination. Current Osteoporosis Reports. 2017;**15**:343-352. DOI: 10.1007/s11914-017-0376-x

[82] Recker RR, Marin F, Ish-Shalom S, et al. Comparative effects of teriparatide and strontium ranelate on bone biopsies and biochemical markers of bone turnover in postmenopausal women with osteoporosis. Journal of Bone and Mineral Research. 2009;**24**:1358-1368. DOI: 10.1359/jbmr.090315

[83] Krege JH, Lane NE, Harris JM, Miller PD. PINP as a biological response marker during teriparatide treatment for osteoporosis. Osteoporosis International. 2014;**25**:2159-2171. DOI: 10.1007/s00198-014-2646-0

[84] Glover SJ, Eastell R, McCloskey EV, Rogers A, Garnero P, Lowery J, et al. Rapid and robust response of biochemical markers of bone formation to teriparatide therapy. Bone. 2009;**45**:1053-1058. DOI: 10.1016/j.bone.2009.07.091

[85] Farahmand P, Marin F, Hawkins F, et al. Early changes in biochemical markers of bone formation during teriparatide therapy correlate with improvements in vertebral strength in men with glucocorticoid-induced osteoporosis. Osteoporosis International. 2013;**24**:2971-2981. DOI: 10.1007/s00198-013-2379-5

[86] McClung MR, Grauer A, Boonen S, et al. Romosozumab in postmenopausal women with low bone mineral density. The New England Journal of Medicine. 2014;**370**:412-420. DOI: 10.1056/NEJMoa1305224

[87] Cosman F, Crittenden DB, Adachi JD, et al. Romosozumab treatment in postmenopausal women with osteoporosis. The New England Journal of Medicine. 2016;**375**:1532-1543. DOI: 10.1056/NEJMoa1607948

[88] Saag KG, Petersen J, Brandi ML, Karaplis AC, Lorentzon M, Thomas T, et al. Romosozumab or alendronate for fracture prevention in women with osteoporosis. The New England Journal of Medicine. 2017;**377**:1417-1427. DOI: 10.1056/NEJMoa1708322

[89] Diez-Perez A, Gonzalez-Macias J. Inadequate responders to osteoporosis treatment: Proposal for an operational definition. Osteoporosis International. 2008;**19**:1511-1516. DOI: 10.1007/s00198-008-0659-2

[90] Sarkar S, Mitlak BH, Wong M, Stock JL, Black DM, Harper KD.

Relationships between bone mineral density and incident vertebral fracture risk with raloxifene therapy. Journal of Bone and Mineral Research. 2002;**17**:1-10. DOI: 10.1359/jbmr.2002.17.1.1

[91] Khosla S. Surrogates for fracture endpoints in clinical trials. Journal of Bone and Mineral Research. 2003;**18**:1146-1149. DOI: 10.1359/jbmr.2003.18.6.1146

[92] Diez-Perez A, Adachi JD, Agnusdei D, et al. Treatment failure in osteoporosis. Osteoporosis International. 2012;**23**:2769-2774. DOI: 10.1007/s00198-012-2093-8

[93] Vasikaran S, Eastell R, Bruyere O, et al. Markers of bone turnover for the prediction of fracture risk and monitoring of osteoporosis treatment: A need for international reference standards. Osteoporosis International. 2011;**22**:391-420. DOI: 10.1007/s00198-010-1501-1

[94] Szulc P. The role of bone turnover markers in monitoring treatment in postmenopausal osteoporosis. Clinical Biochemistry. 2012;**45**:907-919. DOI: 10.1016/j.clinbiochem.2012.01.022

[95] Delmas PD, Munoz F, Black DM, et al. Effects of yearly zoledronic acid 5 mg on bone turnover markers and relation of PINP with fracture reduction in postmenopausal women with osteoporosis. Journal of Bone and Mineral Research. 2009;**24**:1544-1551. DOI: 10.1359/jbmr.090310

[96] Bauer DC, Black DM, Garnero P, Hochberg M, Ott S, Orloff J, et al. Change in bone turnover and hip, non-spine, and vertebral fracture in alendronate-treated women: The fracture intervention trial. Journal of Bone and Mineral Research. 2004;**19**:1250-1258. DOI: 10.1359/JBMR.040512

[97] Ameis A, Randhawa K, Yu H, et al. The global spine care initiative: A review of reviews and recommendations for the non-invasive management of acute osteoporotic vertebral compression fracture pain in low- and middle-income communities. European Spine Journal. 2018;**27**:861-869. DOI: 10.1007/s00586-017-5273-6

[98] Stadhouder A, Buskens E, Vergroesen DA, Fidler MW, de Nies F, Oner FC. Nonoperative treatment of thoracic and lumbar spine fractures: A prospective randomized study of different treatment options. Journal of Orthopaedic Trauma. 2009;**23**:588-594. DOI: 10.1097/BOT.0b013e3181a18728

[99] Kato T, Inose H, Ichimura S, et al. Comparison of rigid and soft-brace treatments for acute osteoporotic vertebral compression fracture: A prospective, randomized, multicenter study. Journal of Clinical Medicine. 2019;**8**:198. DOI: 10.3390/jcm8020198

[100] Klazen CA, Verhaar HJ, Lohle PN, Lampmann LE, Juttmann JR, Schoemaker MC, et al. Clinical course of pain in acute osteoporotic vertebral compression fractures. Journal of Vascular and Interventional Radiology. 2010;**21**:1405-1409. DOI: 10.1016/j.jvir.2010.05.018

[101] Venmans A, Klazen CA, Lohle PN, Mali WP, van Rooij WJ. Natural history of pain in patients with conservatively treated osteoporotic vertebral compression fractures: Results from VERTOS II. AJNR. American Journal of Neuroradiology. 2012;**33**:519-521. DOI: 10.3174/ajnr.A2817

[102] Takahashi S, Hoshino M, Takayama K, et al. The natural course of the paravertebral muscles after the onset of osteoporotic vertebral fracture. Osteoporosis International.

2020;**31**:1089-1095. DOI: 10.1007/s00198-020-05338-8

[103] Zhang J, He X, Fan Y, Du J, Hao D. Risk factors for conservative treatment failure in acute osteoporotic vertebral compression fractures (OVCFs). Archives of Osteoporosis. 2019;**14**:24. DOI: 10.1007/s11657-019-0563-8

[104] Muratore M, Ferrera A, Masse A, Bistolfi A. Osteoporotic vertebral fractures: Predictive factors for conservative treatment failure. A systematic review. European Spine Journal. 2018;**27**:2565-2576. DOI: 10.1007/s00586-017-5340-z

[105] Inose H, Kato T, Ichimura S, et al. Risk factors of nonunion after acute osteoporotic vertebral fractures: A prospective multicenter cohort study. Spine (Phila Pa 1976). 2020;**45**:895-902. DOI: 10.1097/BRS.0000000000003413

[106] Hinde K, Maingard J, Hirsch JA, Phan K, Asadi H, Chandra RV. Mortality outcomes of vertebral augmentation (vertebroplasty and/or balloon kyphoplasty) for osteoporotic vertebral compression fractures: A systematic review and meta-analysis. Radiology. 2020;**295**:96-103. DOI: 10.1148/radiol.2020191294

[107] Tsoumakidou G, Too CW, Koch G, Caudrelier J, Cazzato RL, Garnon J, et al. CIRSE guidelines on percutaneous vertebral augmentation. Cardiovascular and Interventional Radiology. 2017;**40**:331-342. DOI: 10.1007/s00270-017-1574-8

[108] Hayashi T, Maeda T, Masuda M, Ueta T, Shiba K. Morphology of the injured posterior wall causing spinal canal encroachment in osteoporotic vertebral fractures. The Spine Journal. 2016;**16**:946-950. DOI: 10.1016/j.spinee.2016.03.021

[109] Morghen I, Borrelli M, Saletti A, Zoppellari R. Percutaneous vertebroplasty and spinal cord compression: A case report. Journal of Radiological Case Report. 2009;**3**:17-20

[110] Morris O, Mathai J, Weller K. Polymethylmethacrylate pulmonary embolism following kyphoplasty. Clinical Practicing Cases Emergency Medicine. 2019;**3**:226-228

[111] Kim YY, Rhyu KW. Recompression of vertebral body after balloon kyphoplasty for osteoporotic vertebral compression fracture. European Spine Journal. 2010;**19**:1907-1912. DOI: 10.1007/s00586-010-1479-6

[112] Li YX, Guo DQ, Zhang SC, Liang YK, Mo GY, Li DX, et al. Risk factor analysis for re-collapse of cemented vertebrae after percutaneous vertebroplasty (PVP) or percutaneous kyphoplasty (PKP). International Orthopaedics. 2018;**42**:2131-2139. DOI: 10.1007/s00264-018-3838-6

[113] Anselmetti GC, Zoarski G, Manca A, Masala S, Eminefendic H, Russo F, et al. Percutaneous vertebroplasty and bone cement leakage: Clinical experience with a new high-viscosity bone cement and delivery system for vertebral augmentation in benign and malignant compression fractures. Cardiovascular and Interventional Radiology. 2008;**31**:937-947. DOI: 10.1007/s00270-008-9324-6

[114] Yu WB, Jiang XB, Liang D, Xu WX, Ye LQ, Wang J. Risk factors and score for recollapse of the augmented vertebrae after percutaneous vertebroplasty in osteoporotic vertebral compression fractures. Osteoporosis International. 2018;**30**:423-430. DOI: 10.1007/s00198-018-4754-8

[115] Mudano AS, Bian J, Cope JU, et al. Vertebroplasty and kyphoplasty

are associated with an increased risk of secondary vertebral compression fractures: A population-based cohort study. Osteoporosis International. 2009;**20**:819-826. DOI: 10.1007/s00198-008-0745-5

[116] Ebeling PR, Akesson K, Bauer DC, et al. The efficacy and safety of vertebral augmentation: A second ASBMR task force report. Journal of Bone and Mineral Research. 2019;**34**:3-21. DOI: 10.1002/jbmr.3653

[117] Dyer O. Vertebral augmentation in osteoporosis: Common procedures for spinal fractures show no benefit. BMJ. 2019;**364**:l515. DOI: 10.1136/bmj.l515

[118] Clark W, Bird P, Gonski P, Diamond TH, Smerdely P, McNeil HP, et al. Safety and efficacy of vertebroplasty for acute painful osteoporotic fractures (VAPOUR): A multicentre, randomised, double-blind, placebo-controlled trial. Lancet. 2016;**388**:1408-1416. DOI: 10.1016/S0140-6736(16)31341-1

[119] Buchbinder R, Johnston RV, Rischin KJ, Homik J, Jones CA, Golmohammadi K, et al. Percutaneous vertebroplasty for osteoporotic vertebral compression fracture. Cochrane Database of Systematic Reviews. 2018;**4**:CD006349. DOI: 10.1002/14651858.CD006349.pub3

[120] Buchbinder R, Busija L. Why we should stop performing vertebroplasties for osteoporotic spinal fractures. Internal Medicine Journal. 2019;**49**:1367-1371. DOI: 10.1111/imj.14628

[121] Zhao Y, Xue R, Shi N, Xue Y, Zong Y, Lin W, et al. Aggravation of spinal cord compromise following new osteoporotic vertebral compression fracture prevented by teriparatide in patients with surgical contraindications. Osteoporosis International. 2016;**27**:3309-3317. DOI: 10.1007/s00198-016-3651-2

[122] Omi H, Yokoyama T, Ono A, Numasawa T, Wada K, Fujisawa Y. Can MRI predict subsequent pseudarthrosis resulting from osteoporotic thoracolumbar vertebral fractures? European Spine Journal. 2014;**23**:2705-2710. DOI: 10.1007/s00586-014-3490-9

[123] Ma Y, Wu X, Xiao X, Ma Y, Feng L, Yan W, et al. Effects of teriparatide versus percutaneous vertebroplasty on pain relief, quality of life and cost-effectiveness in postmenopausal females with acute osteoporotic vertebral compression fracture: A prospective cohort study. Bone. 2020;**131**:115154. DOI: 10.1016/j.bone.2019.115154

[124] Ha KY, Park KS, Kim SI, Kim YH. Does bisphosphonate-based anti-osteoporosis medication affect osteoporotic spinal fracture healing? Osteoporosis International. 2016;**27**:483-488. DOI: 10.1007/s00198-015-3243-6

[125] Min H-K, Ahn J-H, Ha K-Y, et al. Effects of anti-osteoporosis medications on radiological and clinical results after acute osteoporotic spinal fractures: A retrospective analysis of prospectively designed study. Osteoporosis International. 2019;**30**:2249-2256

[126] Iwata A, Kanayama M, Oha F, Hashimoto T, Iwasaki N. Effect of teriparatide (rh-PTH 1-34) versus bisphosphonate on the healing of osteoporotic vertebral compression fracture: A retrospective comparative study. BMC Musculoskeletal Disorders. 2017;**18**:148. DOI: 10.1186/s12891-017-1509-1

[127] Gou P, Wang Z, Zhao Z, Wang Y, Jiang Y, Xue Y. Restoration of the intravertebral stability in Kummell's disease following the treatment of

severe postmenopausal osteoporosis by 1-34PTH-a retrospective study. Osteoporosis International. 2021;**32**:1451-1459. DOI: 10.1007/s00198-020-05761-x

[128] Gou P, Jing W, Zhou J, Wang R, Wang Z, Chang F, et al. Magnetic resonance imaging negative spine trauma followed by a delayed intravertebral vacuum cleft-Kummell's disease: A case report and literature review. Orthopaedic Surgery. 2023;**15**:366-370. DOI: 10.1111/os.13559

[129] Kim DY, Lee SH, Jang JS, Chung SK, Lee HY. Intravertebral vacuum phenomenon in osteoporotic compression fracture: Report of 67 cases with quantitative evaluation of intravertebral instability. Journal of Neurosurgery. 2004;**100**:24-31. DOI: 10.3171/spi.2004.100.1.0024

[130] McKiernan F, Faciszewski T. Intravertebral clefts in osteoporotic vertebral compression fractures. Arthritis and Rheumatism. 2003;**48**:1414-1419. DOI: 10.1002/art.10984

[131] Tsujio T, Nakamura H, Terai H, et al. Characteristic radiographic or magnetic resonance images of fresh osteoporotic vertebral fractures predicting potential risk for nonunion: A prospective multicenter study. Spine (Phila Pa 1976). 2011;**36**:1229-1235. DOI: 10.1097/BRS.0b013e3181f29e8d

[132] Gou PG, Zhao ZH, Zhou JM, Ren LH, Wang XY, Mu YF, et al. Vertebral collapse prevented following teriparatide treatment in postmenopausal Kummell's disease patients with severe osteoporosis. Orthopaedic Surgery. 2021;**13**:506-516. DOI: 10.1111/os.12959

[133] Diamond T, Clark W, Kumar S. Histomorphometric analysis of fracture healing cascade in acute osteoporotic vertebral body fractures. Bone. 2007;**40**:775-780. DOI: 10.1016/j.bone.2006.10.009

[134] Formica M, Zanirato A, Cavagnaro L, Basso M, Divano S, Lamartina C, et al. Vertebral body osteonecrosis: Proposal of a treatment-oriented classification system. European Spine Journal. 2018;**27**:190-197. DOI: 10.1007/s00586-018-5600-6

[135] Yang H, Pan J, Wang G. A review of osteoporotic vertebral fracture nonunion management. Spine (Phila Pa 1976). 2014;**39**:B4-B6. DOI: 10.1097/BRS.0000000000000538

[136] Laredo JD. Expert's comment concerning grand rounds case entitled "Kummell's disease: Delayed post-traumatic osteonecrosis of the vertebral body" (by Ma R, Chow R, Shen FH). European Spine Journal. 2010;**19**:1071-1072. DOI: 10.1007/s00586-009-1204-5

[137] Matzaroglou C, Georgiou CS, Wilke HJ, Assimakopoulos K, Karageorgos A, Konstantinou D, et al. Kümmell's disease: Is ischemic necrosis or vertebral "microcracking" the first step in the sequence? Medical Hypotheses. 2013;**80**:505. DOI: 10.1016/j.mehy.2012.12.003

[138] Formica M, Basso M, Cavagnaro L, Formica C, Zanirato A, Felli L. Kümmell's disease: Illustrative case for definition criteria. The Spine Journal. 2016;**16**:e707-e708. DOI: 10.1016/j.spinee.2016.03.035

[139] Nakamae T, Fujimoto Y, Yamada K, Takata H, Shimbo T, Tsuchida Y. Percutaneous vertebroplasty for osteoporotic vertebral compression fracture with intravertebral cleft associated with delayed neurologic deficit. European Spine Journal. 2013;**22**:1624-1632. DOI: 10.1007/s00586-013-2686-8

[140] Kawaguchi S et al. Symptomatic relevance of intravertebral cleft in patients with osteoporotic vertebral fracture. Journal of Neurosurgery: Spine. 2010;**13**:267-275. DOI: 10.3171/2010.3.SPINE09364

Chapter 2

Targeting "Immunoporosis" as a Novel Concept of Immunotherapy in the Management and Treatment of Osteoporosis

Vardhan Pol, Taranjeet Kaur, Asha Bhardwaj, Leena Sapra, Sumedha Yadav and Rupesh K. Srivastava

Abstract

Osteoporosis is a skeleton disease characterized by low bone mass, bone tissue deterioration, and alterations in bone microarchitecture. It is estimated that there are more than 500 million patients worldwide who suffer from osteoporosis-related fractures. There are several risk factors for osteoporosis. These comprise common risk factors like aging and steroid deficiency, as well as specific risk factors such as glucocorticoid use, decreased bone quality, and modifications in bone microarchitecture. However, the pivotal role of the immune system in osteoporosis was initially sidelined in the pathophysiology of osteoporosis but has gained much attention in recent years. Current discoveries have highlighted the existence of a vast network of communication between bone and the immune system in the maintenance of bone homeostasis. Moreover, it is observed that the majority of first-line therapies currently used to treat osteoporosis have immunomodulatory potential thereby preventing bone resorption by regulating the "Immunoporotic axis." Therefore, these findings would potentially lead to a dramatic shift in the treatment modalities for the management of inflammatory bone loss observed in osteoporosis. To emphasize the crucial role of the immune system in the pathology of osteoporosis, our group coined the term "Immunoporosis" in 2018. In this chapter, we will comprehensively review the pivotal role of the immune system in the pathophysiology of osteoporosis. Furthermore, we will discuss several novel immunomodulatory strategies that can be exploited for the management and prevention of osteoporosis.

Keywords: osteoporosis, immunoporosis, immunotherapy, T cells, B cells, gut microbiota, probiotics

1. Introduction

Bone is a connective tissue that consists of two main components: extracellular matrix and cellular component. The extracellular matrix comprises organic components such as collagen type 1 fibrils and non-collagenous glycoproteins and proteoglycans, and inorganic components calcium and phosphate carbonate which are organized as hydroxyapatite crystals. The cellular component includes the bone cells (osteoclasts, osteoblasts, and osteocytes) which drive the process of bone remodeling as each cell has its distinct function.

Osteoblasts are anabolic cells that are derived from pluripotent bone mesenchymal stem cells (BMSCs). They are regarded as "Bone Forming Cells" that are cuboidal in shape when present in active form. Osteoblast differentiation from MSCs is genetically controlled by the expression of many genes, such as runt-related transcription factor-2 (Runx2), distal-less homeobox-5 (Dlx5), and osterix (Osx), etc. [1]. Upon aging, the osteoblasts can either undergo apoptosis or transform into osteocytes and bone-lining cells. The bone lining cells depict the resting phase in the bone remodeling process. The prominent functions of osteoblasts are the synthesis of proteins comprising the extracellular matrix, the regulation of osteoclasts via paracrine signaling, and bone matrix mineralization.

Osteoclasts are bone-eating multinucleated large cells that are formed from colony-forming unit-macrophage (CFU-M) lineage progenitors. Macrophage colony-stimulating factor (MCSF) and receptor activator of nuclear factor kappa-B ligand (RANKL) are crucial regulators of osteoclast differentiation. While RANKL enhances the differentiation of progenitors into osteoclasts, MCSF encourages the proliferation and survival of osteoclast progenitors. The role of osteoblasts in osteoclast differentiation and proliferation is associated with the expression of MCSF and RANKL. The resorption by osteoclasts is mediated by dissolving the hydroxyapatite crystals due to the acidification of resorption lacunae which eventually release calcium, minerals, and growth factors residing in the bone matrix.

The entrapped osteoblasts that are embedded in bone matrix are called osteocytes. They are regarded as the most mature form of osteoblasts and have a peculiar role in regulating bone remodeling. Osteocytes have mechanical stress sensors and respond to them via secretion of insulin-like growth factor 1 (IGF-1). The entrapment of osteocytes is essential for their growth and occurs due to the secretion of chemicals in response to mechanical stress only. Bone formation and resorption are also under the influence of osteocytes in response to external mechanical stimuli. Osteocytes have a distinctive spider-like morphology due to the presence of branched cellular processes that form a network of interconnected canaliculi and permit cell-to-cell communication via gap junctions. Upon maturation, the osteoblastic surface markers are lost, while osteocytes gain specific markers namely dentin matrix acidic phosphoprotein (DMP)-1 and Sclerostin (sost). A study on sost-deficient mice suggests that sclerostin negatively regulates osteoblast differentiation via the canonical Wnt pathway and hence controls bone formation [2]. Additionally, osteocytes maintain mineral homeostasis by expressing RANKL expression resulting in osteoclast activity during high calcium demand.

The dynamic process of bone remodeling requires several interactions between osteoblasts and osteoclasts. Bone remodeling preserves the structure of the bone and constantly swaps out the old bone for a new one. Several skeleton malformations are caused by abnormalities in the bone remodeling process. The intricate process of bone remodeling is controlled by several biochemical and mechanical factors. Important elements that play a role in bone regulation are parathyroid hormone (PTH), estrogen, thyroid hormone and glucocorticoids, IGFs, prostaglandins, and bone morphogenetic proteins (BMPs) and vitamin D. Another crucial factor that has a significant role in the regulation of bone health is the immune system. Recent research has shown that the immune and skeleton system actively interacts with one another. Osteoimmunology is a novel branch of immunology that deals with the intricate link between the bone and the immune system [3]. According to experimental data, pro-inflammatory cytokines such as interleukin (IL)-1, IL-6, and tumor necrosis factor (TNF)-α are detrimental to the bone. These discoveries paved the way for the emergence of a distinct discipline known as "Immunoporosis," or the immunology of osteoporosis, which was named by our group in 2018. In clinical applications, understanding immunology is more crucial than ever for the treatment and management of osteoporosis.

This chapter discussed in particular the role of the immune system in osteoporosis i.e., Immunoporosis. Additionally, we suggest that in the long run, focusing on the Immunoporotic-nexus would be a much better immunotherapeutic approach to managing and treating the inflammatory bone loss seen in osteoporosis.

2. Osteoporosis

Osteoporosis is a disease of the bone in which enhanced bone loss, low bone mineral density (BMD), and increased risk of fractures are observed. This bone loss is caused due to many factors. Some of these include dietary intake, smoking, genetics, etc. Mainly post-menopausal women are at a greater risk of suffering from osteoporosis, this is because the hormone estrogen offers an osteoprotective role as it increases osteoclast apoptosis. Estrogen deficiency in post-menopausal women thus leads to osteoporosis. It can occur in males as well. It has affected nearly 500 million people worldwide [4]. This disease is further classified into primary and secondary osteoporosis. Primary osteoporosis is of two types i.e., type 1 (known as post-menopausal osteoporosis) and type 2 (known as senile osteoporosis). Secondary osteoporosis is caused due to certain defined etiological mechanisms. These mechanisms can be ranging from lifestyle factors like excessive smoking, and alcohol consumption to endocrine disorders like hypogonadism, diabetes, etc. The use of drugs like methotrexate and glucocorticoids is also linked with secondary osteoporosis [5]. Often the disease is undetected and remains silent until it is manifested in the form of a fracture. These fractures occur most commonly at the hip, leading to loss of mobility. The primary diagnostic measure for the screening of osteoporosis is the T score obtained by the dual-energy x-ray absorptiometry (DEXA) scan. A score of 2.5 or any score lower than 2.5 marks osteoporosis [4]. As it is now a well-established fact that there is an appraisable interplay between the bone and the skeletal system further sections of this chapter emphasized the immunology of osteoporosis i.e., Immunoporosis.

3. Immunoporosis: the role of the immune system in osteoporosis

In 2002, Osteoimmunology was established as a novel field in the sciences of immunology to study the interaction between the immune system and the skeletal system. In 2018, our group coined the term "Immunoporosis" and highlighted the importance of the "Immune-skeletal" interface in the development of osteoporosis. Cells of the immune system, mainly lymphocytes, have a profound impact on the skeletal system. These cells can either enhance the activity of osteoclasts and lead to more bone resorption or inhibit the activity of osteoclasts, leading to more bone formation. Immune cells carry out this function by the secretion of certain factors, which are known as cytokines. Cells of the lymphoid lineage, mainly subsets of $CD4^+$

T helper cells, B cells, and regulatory B cells (Bregs) have a profound impact on the bone. In addition, cells of the innate immune system also play a crucial role in osteoporosis. In further sections, we will describe the role of innate and adaptive immune cells in the pathophysiology of osteoporosis (**Figure 1**).

3.1 Role of innate immune cells in osteoporosis

Innate immune cells include dendritic cells (DCs), mast cells, eosinophils, basophils, neutrophils, monocytes, macrophages, and innate lymphoid cells (ILCs), etc. Out of these cells, DCs, monocytes, and macrophages have been reported to enhance osteoclast differentiation. Also, these cells, including osteoclasts are derived from a common progenitor. DCs are precursors of osteoclasts and can develop into fully functional multi-nucleated osteoclasts. It has been reported that when $CD11c^+$ DCs interact with $CD4^+$ T cells, they develop into multinucleated osteoclasts [6]. Classical and intermediate monocytes can also differentiate into functional osteoclasts; however, their differentiation depends on the inflammatory conditions. Under physiological conditions, classical monocytes develop into osteoclasts whereas under inflammatory conditions intermediate monocytes develop into osteoclasts. The role of macrophages in bone remodeling is still under investigation. A study carried out by Yamaguchi et al. demonstrated that upon induction with lipopolysaccharide (LPS) and interferon (IFN)-γ M1 macrophages suppressed RANKL-dependent osteoclastogenesis. However, the same results were not observed with M2 macrophages [7]. Another study also reported that M2 macrophages have better osteoclast-forming capabilities than M1 macrophages [8]. Some studies have also correlated allergy with increased bone loss. Mast cells are known to secrete histamine, it has been reported that histamine aids in osteoclastogenesis by directly acting on osteoclasts [9]. Also, a high number of mast cells have been reported in post-menopausal osteoporotic patients. Eosinophils and basophils are also actively involved in allergic inflammation. The major cytokines observed during allergy are IL-31 and IL-33. IL-31 is increased in post-menopausal osteoporotic patients with low BMD [10]. IL-33 on the other hand has an inhibitory effect on osteoclast differentiation, by the release of IL-10 [11].

Natural killer (NK) cells play a crucial role in tumor immunity and protect virus-infected cells. Interesting findings about these cells have been reported in patients suffering from rheumatoid arthritis (RA). Soderstom et al. reported that NK cells produce MCSF and RANKL and promote osteoclast differentiation [12]. However, in 2015, the same group reported that NK cells can inhibit osteoclastogenesis when they get activated by IL-15. Interestingly, IL-15 has been reported to have a dual role. It can promote the apoptosis of osteoclasts as well as osteoblasts [13, 14].

ILCs are classified into three groups i.e., ILC1, ILC2, and ILC3. These cells are mirror images of the T helper subset cells (Th1, Th2, and Th17) and just like them, are dependent on the master transcription factors T-bet, GATA-3, and RORγt and IFN-γ, IL-4, and IL-17 are moreover their distinguishing cytokines [4]. It has been reported that ILCs produce RANKL and might lead to enhanced osteoclast development. ILC1, via the release of IFN-γ, might regulate the bone remodeling process. ILC2 can also release IL-4 and IL-13, thereby offering an osteoprotective role. ILC3 is similar to Th17 cells. They secrete IL-17, which has been associated with increased osteoclast differentiation and therefore might promote bone loss. However, further studies are required to explore the role of ILCs in the progression of osteoporosis. Collectively, these findings suggest that developing strategies that target the innate immune system might be beneficial in the management and treatment of osteoporosis.

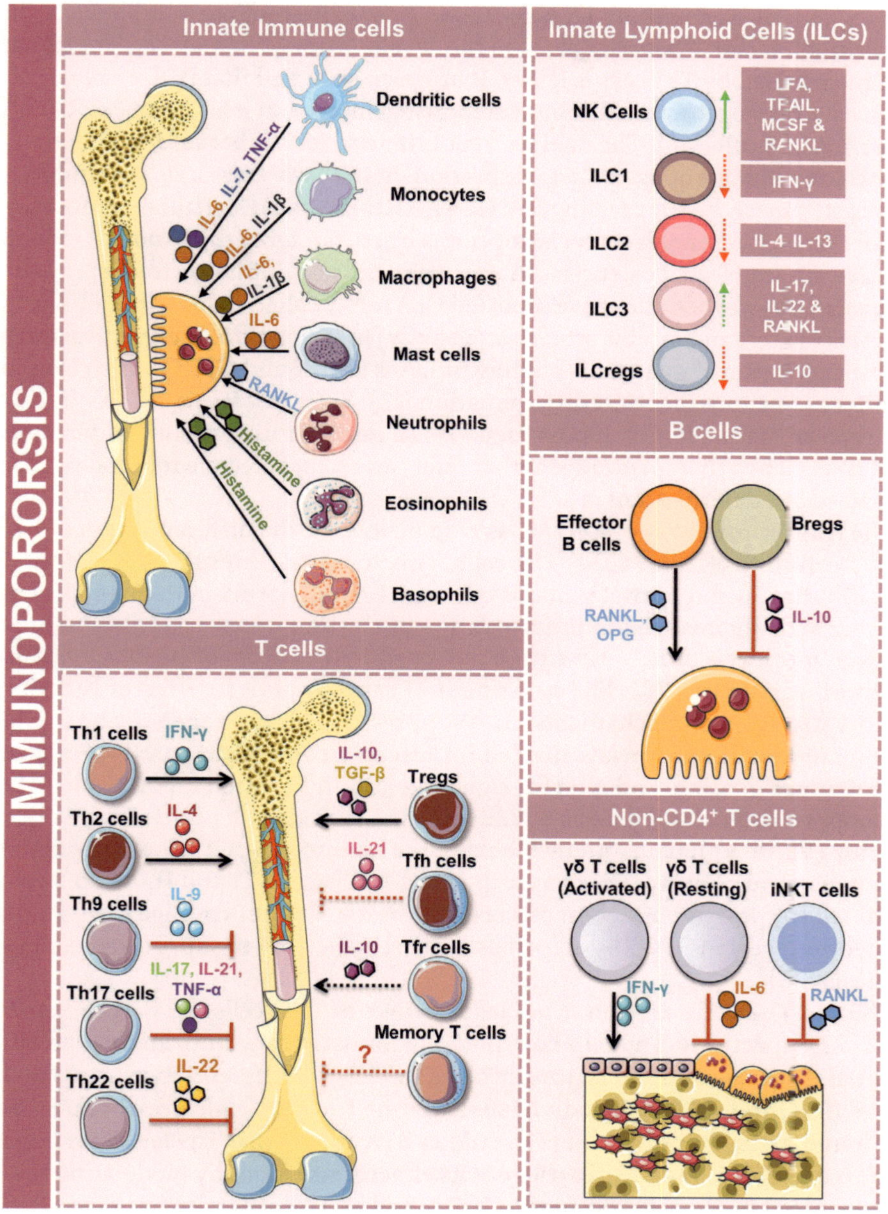

Figure 1.
Role of immune system in osteoporosis i.e., Immunoporosis. Schematic diagram representing the role of different immune cells in the pathophysiology of osteoporosis.

3.2 Role of the adaptive immune system in osteoporosis

3.2.1 T helper cells

A subset of $CD4^+$ lymphoid cells is known as T helper cells. They are divided into the Th1, Th2, Th17, Th9, Th22, T-regulatory cells (Tregs), T-follicular helper cells (Tfh), and memory T cells based on surface markers, their cytokine profile, and transcription factors.

Upon stimulation with IL-12, naïve CD4⁺ T cells differentiate into Th1 cells. The transcription factor T-bet is involved in the development of this subset. The signature cytokine released by Th1 cells is IFN-γ. It has been observed that IFN-γ has a dual role in osteoclastogenesis. It inhibits osteoclastogenesis, but it also induces RANKL expression in T cells [15]. The dual nature of this cytokine is because its effect depends on the stage of osteoclast maturation. In the early stages, IFN-γ inhibits osteoclastogenesis by suppressing RANK-RANKL-mediated signaling. Interestingly, in later stages, it promotes osteoclastogenesis by encouraging the fusion of monocytes to form multi-nucleated osteoclasts. It can carry out its inhibitory effect via other mechanisms as well. Studies have reported that IFN-γ collaborates with toll-like receptors (TLRs) and inhibit osteoclastogenesis [16]. This cytokine can also upregulate the expression of guanylate-binding proteins (GBP2 and GBP5) which have an inhibitory effect on osteoclast differentiation [17]. Since low levels of IFN-γ have also been reported in the serum of post-menopausal osteoporotic patients, this cytokine could be used as a therapeutic agent that offers an osteoprotective role and potentially alleviates bone deterioration [4].

The transcription factor GATA-3 is responsible for the differentiation of naïve $CD4^+$ T cells into effector $CD4^+$ Th2 cells. This subset secretes IL-4, IL-5, and IL-13. Studies have reported that out of these three signature cytokines, IL-4 and IL-13 are actively involved in the regulation of the Immunoporotic axis. Similar to IFN-γ, low levels of IL-4 have been observed in the serum of post-menopausal osteoporotic patients [18]. The cytokine IL-4 can carry out its effector functions via a diverse array of mechanisms. IL-4 suppresses osteoclastogenesis by inhibiting three main signaling pathways needed for osteoclast function i.e., NF-κB signaling, calcium signaling, and NFATc1 signaling [19]. It has been reported that IL-4 can suppress osteoclastogenesis by inducing the peroxisome proliferator-activated receptor (PPAR-γ) ligand and by blocking the interaction of TNF-α with signal transducers and activators of transcription (STAT)-6. IL-13 and IL-4 can have a combined suppressive effect on osteoclastogenesis. They encourage the production of osteoprotegerin (OPG) by osteoblasts, thereby leading to suppressed osteoclastogenesis [20].

Th9 and Th22 cells are said to be close relatives of Th17 cells and they secrete IL-9 and IL-22 respectively. Th9 cells have both inflammatory and anti-inflammatory potential. The transcription factors involved in Th9 cell differentiation are Foxo-1, STAT6, IRF4, and GATA3. In individuals suffering from RA high levels of IL-9 have been found in the synovial fluid [21]. Studies have shown that Th9 levels are positively correlated with RA. IL-9 also carries out its effector functions by modulating the genes involved in osteoclastogenesis. Th22 cells, like Th9 cells, also promote osteoclast differentiation by the secretion of their signature cytokine IL-22 [22]. However, further research should still be carried out to explore the Immunoporotic potential of these cells in case of osteoporosis.

The transcription factor B cell lymphoma-6/Bcl-6 is involved in the differentiation of Tfh cells. This subset of T cells is involved in B cell development. However, Tfh cells are reported to be highly correlated in RA patients. Ma et al. have observed that these cells promote inflammation in RA by the secretion of cytokine IL-21 [23]. A recently identified T follicular regulatory cell (Tfr), has been reported to have a suppressing effect on the Tfh cells observed in RA patients. A study carried out by Niu et al. in 2018 revealed that the dysregulation of the "Tfh-Tfr" ratio in RA patients is caused due to enhanced IL-6/pSTAT3 signaling [24]. Studies have also shown that estrogen is responsible for inhibiting Tfh activity. Estrogen mediates this activity by suppressing the expression of Bcl-6, which is important in Tfh differentiation [25]. The research on Tfh is still limited and the role of this distinct subset of T cells in osteoporosis can be further explored.

Memory T cells are the surviving population of T cells generated after the pool of antigen-activated effector cells declines in population. The population of memory T cells is maintained by the cytokines IL-7 and IL-15 [26]. Memory T cells are subdivided into further populations. These mainly include central memory T cells, effector memory T cells, and tissue-resident memory T cells. Memory T cells act as a linker between allergy and bone loss. A study reported that Th2 cells increased bone loss in the allergic enteropathy mice model by increasing the population of $CD4^{+}CD44^{hi}CD62L^{lo}$ effector memory T cells. This data might support the hypothesis that there might be an osteoporosis-specific antigen that leads to the development of memory T cells [27].

The balance of Treg and Th17 cells in osteoporosis is the crucial determining factor in the development of this disease. Th17 cells secrete IL-17, which promotes osteoclastogenesis, whereas Tregs secrete IL-10, which is anti-osteoclastogenic in nature. $CD4^{+}CD25^{+}FoxP3^{+}$ Tregs, via secreting IL-10 and transforming growth factor (TGF)-β inhibit osteoclastogenesis [28]. Apart from carrying out their effector functions via cytokines, they can suppress osteoclast differentiation via expressing Cytotoxic T lymphocyte antigen-4 (CTLA-4), an inhibitory ligand, which interacts with CD80/86 on the precursors of osteoclasts [29]. Th17 cells are osteoclastogenic in nature. They secrete inflammatory cytokines like IL-6, IL-17, TNF-α, and RANKL, which further enhance osteoclastogenesis. IL-6 supports osteoclastogenesis as it is reported to help in the conversion of Tregs to Th17 cells. This cross-talk between Tregs and Th17 cells generates the "Treg-Th17" axis, which heavily influences osteoclastogenesis and ultimately bone resorption [30].

3.3 Non-$CD4^{+}$ T cells involved in osteoporosis

γδ T cells (Gamma- Delta T cells) and natural killer T cells have been reported to play a role in certain auto-immune diseases where increased bone loss is observed [31]. Unfortunately, their direct role in osteoporosis is still unknown. Most of the T cells express the αβ receptor on their surface. However, a small subpopulation of T cells (1–5% in peripheral circulation) express the unconventional γδ receptor. The γδ T cells are known to secrete IL-6 and IFN-γ, both of these cytokines harness pro and anti-osteoclastogenic roles [32]. A distinct γδ T cell population which also secretes IL-17 ($\gamma\delta17^{+}$ T cells) has been reported to improve effector functions of the cells from lymphoid and myeloid lineage. Their differentiation is supported by IL-23 and literature suggests that these cells might possess some osteoprotective functions. Unfortunately, no studies to date have investigated the role of $\gamma\delta17^{+}$ T cells in post-menopausal osteoporosis [4].

Invariant Natural killer T cells or iNKT cells can promote osteoclastogenesis in a RANKL-dependent manner. These cells express high levels of RANKL in osteoporotic patients [33]. They can indirectly enhance osteoclastogenesis by activating myeloid DCs and macrophages, which are osteoclast precursors.

3.4 Role of B cells in osteoporosis

B cells are classified into B-1 B cells and B-2 B cells. B-1 B cells are derived from hematopoietic stem cells (HSCs) found in the fetal liver, whereas B-2 B cells are derived from HSCs in the bone marrow. They are further classified as marginal zone and follicular B cells. B cells can directly impact the RANKL/OPG ratio, which is a very important contributing factor in osteoporosis. It has been reported that B cells release RANKL, which promotes not only osteoclastogenesis but also increases the population of B cells. This forms a vicious cycle resulting in bone loss [34, 35]. Studies also report that B cells harm osteoblasts as well. B cells release osteoblast-inhibiting factors which include chemokine ligand (CCL)-3 and TNF that activate NF-κB and ERK signaling in osteoblasts, ultimately leading to dysfunctional osteoblasts [36]. These findings suggest that B cells might be an interesting target for the treatment of osteoporosis.

In the early 2000s, the role of regulatory B cells (Bregs) in the modification of immune responses during inflammatory conditions has been well established. Based on different phenotypic markers, Bregs are further divided into distinct subsets. Studies on murine Bregs and human Bregs have established the fact that Bregs offer an osteoprotective role. Their signature cytokines include IL-10, IL-35, and TGF-β. IL-10 and TGF-β can have a direct impact on the Treg/Th17 balance. Our group has also reported that there is a subsequent decrease in the number of IL-10 secreting Bregs ($CD19^{+}CD1d^{hi}CD5^{+}$) in the osteoporotic mice model [37]. IL-35 secreted by Bregs has also been shown to suppress osteoclastogenesis. IL-35 induces the production of OPG, which is a decoy receptor for RANKL [38]. Therefore, Bregs have a pivotal role in the pathogenesis of osteoporosis.

4. Harnessing immunotherapy for osteoporosis

Therapies for osteoporosis include anti-resorptive and anti-osteoclastogenic drugs. First-line anti-resorptive drugs include bisphosphonates, denosumab, and teriparatide. Bisphosphonates are the most common first-line therapy for osteoporosis. They inhibit osteoclast differentiation [39]. Denosumab is an antibody against RANKL. It is a fully humanized, IgG2 resembling, monoclonal antibody. The administration of denosumab has been shown to reduce bone resorption and enhance trabecular bone microstructure [40]. Teriparatide is a synthetic version of the parathyroid hormone. Intermittent dosage of teriparatide has been shown to enhance osteoblast activity [41]. Apart from their direct effect on the bone cells, it is observed that the majority of first-line therapies for osteoporosis have immunomodulatory potential. Therefore, it is plausible to suggest that these drugs are also inhibiting bone resorption by regulating the "Immunoporotic axis." Below the role of various drugs in regulating the Immunoporotic axis has been explained along with this we have also suggested various novel immunotherapeutics that can be utilized as a treatment modality for osteoporosis by exploiting the immunoporotic axis (**Table 1**) (**Figure 2**).

4.1 Effect of already existing first-line therapies on immunoporotic axis

4.1.1 Bisphosphonates

Bisphosphonates are drugs that inhibit the enzyme farnesyl diphosphate synthase i.e., FPP synthase. This enzyme is responsible for the synthesis of isoprenoid lipids, which further are necessary for the post-translational prenylation of GTPases (mostly of Ras, Rho, and Rab families). Since this enzyme is blocked, the prenylation of the

First Line Therapies		
S. No.	**Therapies**	**Immunoporotic mechanism of Action**
1.	Bisphosphonates	• Regulate the cytokine balance between Tregs and Th17 cells (decrease levels of IL-6, IL-17, and IFN-γ while enhancing the levels of IL-4, IL-10, and TGF-β in plasma). • Regulate γδ T cells (activated)
2.	Teriparatide	• Increase frequency of Tregs
3.	Denosumab	• Prevents interaction of RANKL with RANK receptor
4.	Harmone replacement therapy	• Regulate Treg-Th17 cell axis
Novel Immunotherapeutics		
1.	Phytotherapy	• Regulate Immunoporotic axis (Breg-Treg-Th17 cell axis)
2.	Probiotics	• Regulate Immunoporotic axis (Breg-Treg-Th17 cell axis)
3.	Short-chain fatty acids (SCFAs)	• Induce differentiation of Tregs • Inhibit differentiation of Th17 cells
4.	Bile Acids	• Induce differentiation of Tregs • Inhibit differentiation of Th17 cells
5.	Tryptophan metabolites	• Induce differentiation of Bregs

Table 1.
Role of various first-line therapies and novel immunotherapeutics in regulating the bone health by modulating the immunoporotic axis.

GTPases is inhibited and their function is ultimately blocked. Further, *in-vivo* studies have reported that when bisphosphonates inhibit FPP synthase, the substrates of this enzyme isopentenyl diphosphate (IPP) and dimethylallyl phosphate (DMAPP) accumulate in the cytosol, and by an unknown mechanism, activate a specific subset of γδ T cells (VγVδ2⁺ T cells). It has been reported that IPP and DMAPP are activators of VγVδ2⁺ T cells. These cells also secrete IFN-γ, when treated with zoledronic acid. Therefore, these cells can be a potential target for the treatment of osteoporosis [42]. Apart from exerting their effect on VγVδ2⁺ T cells, bisphosphonates also can modulate the cytokine balance between Th17 cells and Treg cells. According to a study, there was a significant decrease of IL-6, IL-17, and IFN-γ in the plasma levels of osteoporotic patients who received yearly bisphosphonate treatment. There was a significant increase in IL-4, IL-10, and TGF-β plasma levels as well. Since it was earlier mentioned that IFN-γ plays a dual role in the pathophysiology of osteoporosis, this study has not reported the exact correlation of IFN-γ with treated osteoporotic patients. Zoledronic acid inhibits the proliferation of Treg cells *in vitro*. The immunosuppressive functions of Treg cells are thus heavily impaired due to the action of zoledronic acid [43]. A study reported that bisphosphonates can directly lead to the expansion of antibody-producing B cells. This study concludes that bisphosphonates can enhance humoral immune response [44]. However, the effect of bisphosphonates

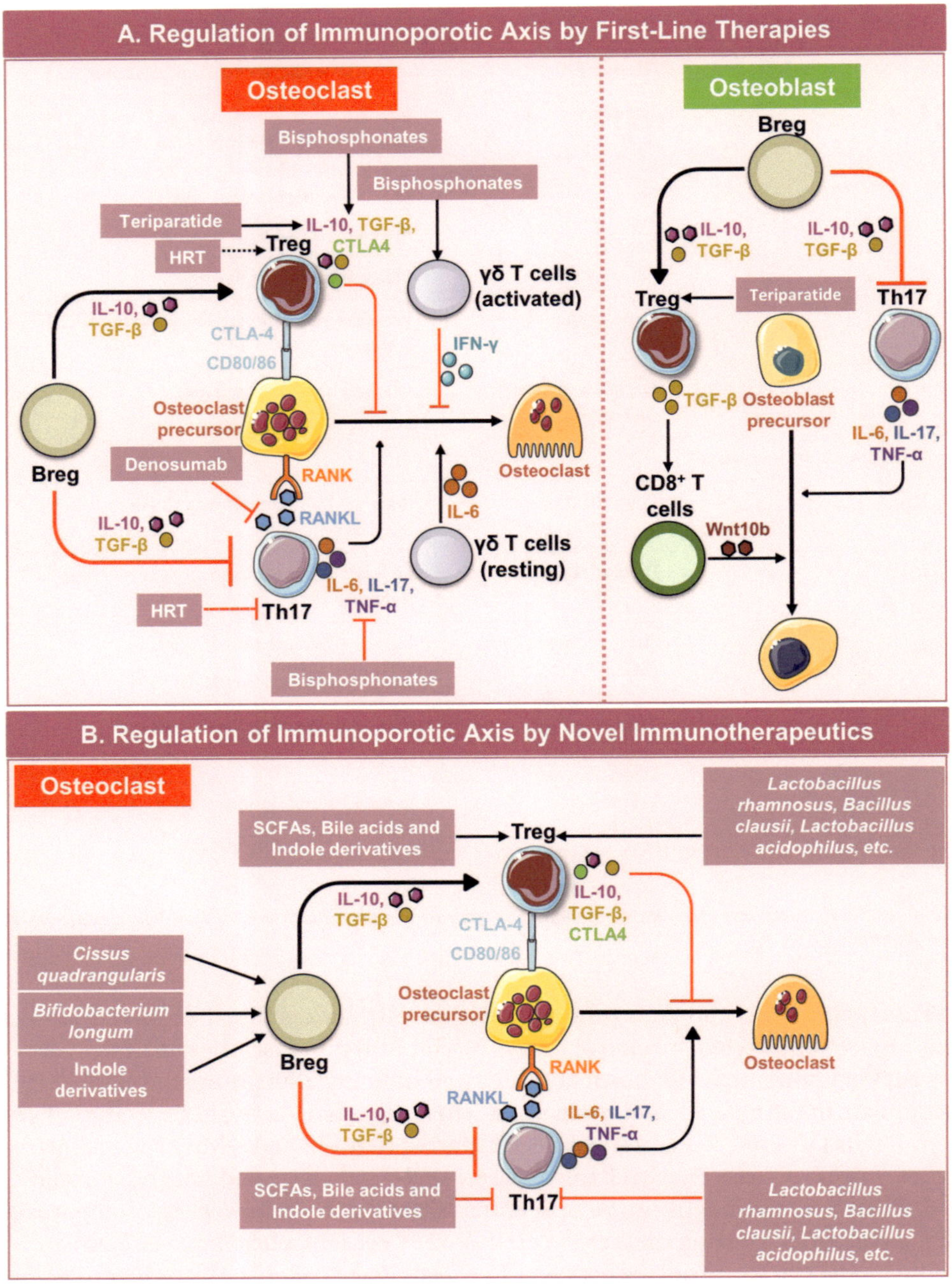

Figure 2.
Role of immune cells in regulating bone remodeling and potential therapeutic checkpoints. (A) Immune cells regulate the activity of osteoclasts and osteoblasts by producing various cytokines. First-line therapies can regulate the bone remodeling by further regulating these immune cells. (B) Various novel immunotherapeutics such as phototherapeutics, probiotics, and their metabolites like short-chain fatty acids (SCFAs), bile acids, and tryptophan metabolites have strong immunomodulatory properties and are observed to regulate the bone remodeling by modulating the immune system.

on Bregs and ultimately on the "Breg-Th17-Treg" axis is still undetermined. Even though studies have shown the effect of bisphosphonates on the immune system, the immune-modulatory properties of these drugs should be further investigated.

4.1.2 Teriparatide

Teriparatide is a synthetic version of the human parathyroid hormone. It is made up of the first 34 amino acids of the parathyroid hormone. It was first approved for medical use in 1987 and later, in November 2002, was approved for the treatment of osteoporosis by the Food and Drug administration (FDA). Unlike bisphosphonates, teriparatide has fewer side effects and can even offer protection against bisphosphonate-related osteonecrosis of the jaw i.e., BRONJ [45]. Teriparatide has an anabolic effect on bone. This synthetic peptide has a direct effect on osteocytes, osteoblasts, and T cells. It is either administered continuously or intermittently. This therapy is therefore known as cPTH or iPTH therapy. iPTH treatment has been reported to reduce the risk of fractures in humans, however, cPTH infusion might harm bone health. It has been reported that cPTH treatment results in cortical bone loss, mainly by activating osteoclast formation [46]. Sclerostin has an inhibitory effect on osteoblast activity and it has been reported that there exists an inverse correlation between sclerostin and PTH levels in healthy women [47]. iPTH treatment leads to the repression of sclerostin and enhances the activity of osteoblasts which results in improved bone health. T cells bearing the receptor for PTH (PPR) act as key mediators in carrying out the effector functions of iPTH. It has been shown that when PTH interacts with the PPR receptor on T cells, Wnt10b signaling is enhanced which lowers the production of sclerostin, whilst increasing osteoblastogenesis [46]. As mentioned earlier, bisphosphonates exert their effect mainly via $CD4^+$ T helper cells. Interestingly, $CD8^+$ T cells are involved in carrying out the effector functions of teriparatide. The engagement of $CD8^+$ T cells became apparent when it was seen that iPTH was unable to show its anabolic effect in the absence of $CD8^+$ T cells. Therefore, literary evidence suggests that Wnt10b, which is an important ligand for osteoblast activity along with $CD8^+$ T cells is important for carrying out the anabolic function of teriparatide [48, 49]. To further support this fact, a study carried out by Terauchi et al. showed that iPTH increased serum levels of osteocalcin (a marker of bone formation) in T cell-reconstituted mice but not in T cell-deficient mice [49]. A similar effect on bone resorption was seen, via observing the serum C-terminal telopeptide of collagen (CTX) levels. The same group also reported that iPTH increased the production of RANKL by both $CD4^+$ T cells and $CD8^+$ T cells [49]. Since RANKL is a known inducer of osteoclastogenesis, the use of iPTH for the treatment of osteoporosis can be questioned. Together these findings establish the cross-talk between the anabolic effects of teriparatide and T cells. Since Tregs are an important component of osteoimmunology, the effect of this synthetic peptide on these subsets can be of immense value. An *in vitro* study carried out by Yu et al. reported that teriparatide did not increase the number of $CD4^+CD25^+FoxP3^+$ T cells in cultures of peripheral blood $CD4^+CD25^+$ T cells. Yu et al. suggest that teriparatide might affect the Treg population via unknown, indirect mechanisms [50]. Although much data is not available on the effect of teriparatide on B lymphocytes, recent studies show that the PPR receptor is important for B cell maturation and function. It has been demonstrated that the loss of PPR on osteoprogenitors leads to impaired B cell maturation and further causes their egress from bone marrow [51]. This finding very much correlates with the fact that T cells also utilize the PPR receptor for enhancing osteoblast activity. These findings together suggest that the teriparatide actively harnesses the adaptive immune system to carry out its anabolic effects on bone, and this crosstalk between teriparatide and cells of the adaptive immune system might be a good candidate for Immunotherapeutics.

4.1.3 Denosumab

Denosumab is a fully humanized monoclonal antibody resembling IgG_2. It has a high affinity for RANKL and its mode of action is similar to the naturally produced RANKL inhibitor OPG. It was manufactured by Amgen, USA, and was approved by FDA for use in 2010. According to Lewiecki yearly use of denosumab marked an increased BMD at the lumbar spine (from 3.0 to 6.7%) and at the hip (from 1.9 to 3.6%). Data from many, phase II randomized studies reveal that denosumab enhances bone health. A significant increase in BMD at the lumbar spine was observed in all the randomized studies [52]. Although no significant effect of denosumab on immune cells was reported. However, Rossini et al. reported that during 1-year administration of denosumab, the number of B cells and $CD4^+$ T cells increased and remained at a higher percentage for 1 year [53]. The RANK receptor, apart from osteoclasts, is also expressed in immune cells which release pro-inflammatory cytokines and are important in mounting an immune response. The inhibition of this system by the use of denosumab has been linked with an increased risk of infections and side effects due to the suppression of the immune system. Even though increased BMD was observed in patients receiving denosumab treatment, the severe risk of infections remains an issue. Therefore, a deeper understanding of the RANK/RANKL/OPG axis can lead to the development of better strategies that harness the Immune-skeletal interface and thus help in the efficient management of osteoporosis.

4.1.4 Anti-sclerostin antibody

Sclerostin is a glycoprotein released by osteocytes that blocks the Wnt signaling needed for osteoblast formation. More sclerostin means less bone formation, which ultimately leads to bone loss. Since sclerostin binds to Wnt molecules, it became an attractive pharmacological target. Eventually, Amgen released romosozumab in 2019 which is a fully humanized monoclonal antibody against sclerostin. It binds to sclerostin and prevents its interaction with Wnt signaling molecules. Wnt then interacts with its transmembrane receptor LRP5/6, which dephosphorylates the protein axin. This leads to the rise of β-catenin, which enhances the transcription of Runx2 and OPG. Ultimately, sclerostin inhibition enhances the Wnt-signaling cascade, which leads to osteoblast differentiation and proliferation [54]. Studies reported that the use of romosozumab led to increased BMD in the lumbar spine, decreased incidence of fractures, and increased cortical bone architecture [55, 56]. When combined with teriparatide and bisphosphonates, a significant increase in BMD at the lumbar spine and hip was also observed. However, no significant difference was observed when romosozumab was combined with denosumab [54]. Another anti-sclerostin antibody, blomosozumab, offered similar results i.e., an increase in BMD and reduced risk of fractures. Unfortunately, the use of romosozumab is associated with adverse side effects as well. It was observed that the use of romosozumab was associated with increased cardiovascular risks [57].

4.1.5 Cathepsin K inhibitors

Cathepsin K is a proteolytic enzyme that belongs to the class of cysteine proteases and is coded by the gene *CstK*. It is abundant in osteoclasts and is highly efficient in cleaving the complex triple helix of type I collagen. Since this enzyme plays a crucial role in bone remodeling, it has been identified as a potential therapeutic target. This rationale has been proven by animal studies. Pennypacker et al. have demonstrated that cathepsin K knockout mice have enhanced bone health i.e., increased BMD, increased trabecular bone, and overall higher bone strength [58]. On the other hand, overexpression of cathepsin K in mice led to increased bone turnover [59]. Some of the most widely used cathepsin K inhibitors are odanacatib, relacatib, and balicatib. Out of all the three drugs, odanacatib has the highest cathepsin K inhibiting potential with very limiting side effects. It has been reported that odanacatib does not have an inhibitory effect on other closely related cathepsins (cathepsin L, S, and V), which are present in different cells and are important for homeostasis [60].

4.1.6 Hormone replacement therapy (HRT)

Estrogen insufficiency is the most common cause of postmenopausal osteoporosis, resulting in rapid bone loss that peaks within the first 2–3 years after menopause. Hormone replacement therapy (HRT) has been considered one of the first-line therapy. HRT replaces hormones that women lose throughout the menopausal transition. To alleviate the symptoms of menopause, conventional HRT contains estrogen and progesterone to mimic hormones produced by the human ovary. It includes only estrogen therapies and estrogen-progesterone or progestin hormone therapy. HRT inhibits not only bone loss and the degeneration of bone microarchitecture but also reduces the risk of fracture by 20–40% at all bone sites. However, the preventive impact of HRT on BMD reduces at an unexpected rate after medication discontinuation, albeit some degree of fracture protection may exist following HRT discontinuation [61]. HRT's osteoprotective and fracture-prevention effects were diminished and non-significant in women over the age of 60. Also, the adverse effects of using HRT include an increased risk of breast cancer, endometrial cancer, blood clots, and stroke with long-term use [62]. There are numerous estrogen medications available, including those produced by the human ovary, such as estradiol and estriol. Conjugated equine estrogen (CEE), the most often prescribed estrogen in the United States, is one of the several estrogenic chemicals [63]. Estrogen is easily absorbed by the gastrointestinal (GI) tract, skin, and mucous membranes. Estrogen has strong immunomodulatory properties and has a role in preventing osteoporosis by influencing the Breg-Treg-Th17 cell axis i.e., the immunoporotic axis [37, 64].

4.2 Novel immunotherapeutics for osteoporosis

As already discussed, most of the currently available first-line therapies have the capability of modulating the immune system and therefore might be preventing bone loss by influencing the immune system. However, these therapies are associated with several side effects and thus there is an urgent need for effective therapeutics with fewer side effects. Below we have suggested some compounds that have shown phenomenal immunomodulatory properties and therefore can be utilized for the prevention and management of osteoporosis (**Figure 2**).

4.2.1 Phytotherapy

Recently, emerging research has shown that many plants and herbs harness immunomodulatory properties. Bioactive compounds from the plants *Moringa oleifera*, *Curcuma longa,* and *Cissus quadrangularis*, modulate the immune system and play a therapeutic role in osteoporosis. Our group has reported that the administration of

C. quadrangularis has a positive effect on bone health, by modulating the immune cells involved in osteoporosis [65]. Sitosterol-3-O-D-glucoside, niazirin, and marumoside A are compounds found in the seeds of *Moringa oleifera*. Ma et al. have reported that all three compounds suppress the secretion of pro-inflammatory cytokines IL-17A and IL-22. The leaves of the same plant also contain a compound quercetin, which inhibits RANKL production and the secretion of IL-17 from Th17 cells. Another such RANKL inhibitor is a compound called 18-glycyrrhetinic acid (isolated from the roots of *Glycrrhiza glabra*), which blocks RANKL-induced osteoclast differentiation [66]. This compound inhibits the interaction of TRAF6 with RANKL, which further prevents the activation of MAPK and NF-κB pathways. Many other plants like *Cucurma longa, Psoralea corylifolia, and Crocus sativus* suppress RANKL-induced osteoclastogenesis [67–71]. Therefore, phytotherapy can be considered an excellent treatment option for osteoporosis however further scientific evidence is required for employing phytotherapy in an osteoporosis` treatment regime.

4.2.2 Probiotics

The probiotics are live non-pathogenic microorganisms that harbor health benefits to individuals when administered in adequate amounts. Numerous bacterial genera, including *Lactobacillus*, *Enterococcus, Bacillus, Escherichia*, and *Bifidobacterium*, have been employed as probiotics due to their advantageous effects. A microbe must exhibit certain traits to be labeled as a probiotic, including the ability to tolerate acid and bile, remain stable in terms of genotype and phenotype, adhere to mucosal surfaces, be resistant to antibiotics, produce antimicrobial substances, and be able to inhibit known pathogens.

Several studies have highlighted the role of probiotics in preventing bone loss by modulating the immune system. In healthy animal model studies, the effect of probiotics was observed to be strain and gender dependent. When *Lactobacillus reuteri* ATCC 6475 was given orally for about 4 weeks to mice, an increased bone mineral density was observed only in male mice. Furthermore, there was enhanced osteocalcin expression as well as an increased rate of bone formation while reduced expression of inflammatory cytokine TNF-α in the jejunum and ileum. In females, under a mild inflammatory state, oral administration of probiotics resulted in enhanced bone density after 8 weeks rather than 4 weeks (as in males). The conclusion from this experiment was that, in healthy conditions, an anti-inflammatory environment is experienced by females which prevented any effect of *L. reuteri* administration. But as soon as a pro-inflammatory environment is induced, the benefactor role of *L. reuteri* can be witnessed [72].

The immune system has a prominent role in regulating bone health and osteoporosis [4, 73, 74]. *Bifidobacterium longum* (BL) via enhancing anti-osteoclastogenic and immunomodulating potential of Bregs ameliorates the bone health in Ovx (ovariectomized) mice [64]. The differentiation and functional activity of RANKL-induced osteoclastogenesis are suppressed by BL in both mouse bone marrow cells and human PBMCs. In comparison to control Bregs, BL-induced Bregs were found to be much more effective at inhibiting osteoclastogenesis and altering the balance of Treg-Th17 cells [64]. Other studies reveal that probiotics like *Lactobacillus rhamnosus*, *Lactobacillus acidophilus,* and *Bacillus clausii* maintain the Tregs-Th17 balance, hence preventing bone loss [75–77]. Therefore, it can be concluded that supplements like probiotics and fermented products can enhance bone health. Hence, probiotics can serve as an adjunct therapy for patients suffering from primary or secondary osteoporosis as they are actively involved in the regulation of the "Breg-Treg-Th17" cell axis.

4.2.3 Postbiotics

The interplay between the immune system, bone, and the gut microbiota is known as the "Gut-Immune-Bone" axis. It is very important in osteoporosis. The immune cells participating in the "Immunoporotic" axis are directly affected by the metabolites secreted from the gut microbiota. Bregs are encouraged to differentiate by a number of gut-associated metabolites (GAMs), including butyrate, 5-hydroxy indole-3-acetic acid (HIAA), acetate, propionate, and pentanoate. These compounds boost the AhR transcription factor's activity, which is essential for Bregs differentiation. So, after their investigation into the effects of probiotics, researchers focused on microbial metabolites such as short-chain fatty acids (SCFAs) like acetate, propionate, butyrate, and tryptophan metabolites, among others. In this chapter, the immunomodulatory capabilities of SCFAs, bile acids, and tryptophan metabolites are covered.

4.2.3.1 Short-chain fatty acids (SCFAs)

SCFAs are widely studied fermented metabolites of gut microbiota that diffuse in the bloodstream and regulate effector functions of distant organs. Butyrate is a histone deacetylase inhibitor and it is known to inhibit osteoclastogenesis. The immune function of SCFAs includes the antimicrobial metabolite production by intestinal macrophages as well as NLR3 inflammasome activation via receptor binding. They also down-regulate the proinflammatory mediators such as Nitric Oxide (NO), IL-6, and IL-12, induced by lipopolysaccharide (LPS) hence, controlling the systemic inflammation. Treg differentiation and proliferation are also controlled by SCFAs with butyrate being the most potent followed by propionate while acetate regulates B cell functions [78]. The negative regulation of osteoclasts by butyrate and propionate occurs via a receptor-independent mechanism along with enhanced glycolysis in osteoclasts which was specified by blocking glycolysis which reverted the anti-osteoclastogenic potential of these SCFAs [79]. A research study by Tyagi et al. reported that butyrate-induced Tregs promote $CD8^+$ T cells to secrete Wnt10b, a bone anabolic Wnt ligand. All these studies suggest that supplementation of SCFAs in patients with osteoporosis can be a novel therapeutic strategy and it can act as an adjunct therapy along with first-line immunotherapies.

4.2.3.2 Bile acids

The primary bile acids, synthesized in the liver and secreted into the duodenum by the host are essential for lipid and glucose metabolism, and confer antibacterial defenses when converted into secondary bile acids by gut microbiota. Cholic acid and chenodeoxycholic acid are two majorly synthesized bile acids in the human liver. The gut microbiota converts cholic acid to deoxycholic acid and lithocholic acid, regarded as secondary bile acids, and has immunomodulatory effects. It has been reported that two derivatives of LCA i.e., 3-oxo-Lithocholic acid and isoallo-Lithocholic acid have been found to affect adaptive immunity. Former has an inhibitory effect on Th17 cells and later influences the enhanced differentiation of T regulatory cells by increasing FoxP3 expression in low TGFβ concentrations via mitochondrial reactive oxygen species (mitoROS) [80, 81]. The enhanced differentiation of Tregs by IsoalloLCA occurs via the nuclear hormone receptor, NR41A. Secondary bile acids induce the immune system to produce anti-inflammatory cytokines in the gastrointestinal tract. Ursodeoxycholic acid, a secondary bile acid has been found to enhance osteoblastogenesis in Saos-2 a human osteosarcoma cell line [82]. A study revealed that targeting bile acid receptors FXR and TGR5 receptors attenuated not only osteoclastogenesis but also enhanced osteoblastogenesis [83]. Further studies need to be done to observe the role of bile acids in osteoporotic patients, either directly or via the immune system. Our group is also exploring the role of secondary bile acids, modified by gut microbiota in the pathophysiology of Osteoporosis.

4.2.3.3 Tryptophan metabolites

Tryptophan, an essential amino acid is catabolized into its derivatives by the gut microbiota that maintains the immune cell homeostasis and function. There are two pathways by which tryptophan is converted to its metabolites, direct pathway which results in indole, tryptamine, indole ethanol (IE), indole lactic acid (ILA), indole propionic acid (IPA), indole acetic acid (IAA), indole aldehyde (IAld), etc. whereas kynurenine and 3-hydroxyanthranilic acid (HAA) are products of Kynurenine pathway. Tryptophan metabolites regulate the differentiation of immune cells through transcription factors such as the aryl hydrocarbon receptor (AhR) that are expressed by immune cells such as macrophages, T-cells, B-cells, ILCs, etc. The tryptophan metabolites control the differentiation and proliferation of Tregs, Bregs, and ILC3 along with anti-inflammatory macrophages. When the AhR ligand binds to its receptor, it translocates from the cytoplasm into the nucleus and forms heterodimers with the nuclear translocator of AhR, and binds to the gene promoter.

Studies reveal that AhR ligands and receptors are potentially involved in the induction of Tregs to produce anti-inflammatory cytokines i.e., IL-10 and IL-22 [84]. The AhR ligands 2,3,7,8-tetrachlorodibenzo-p-dioxin (TCDD) induce Tregs proliferation while 2-(1'H-indolo-3′-carbonyl)-thiazole-4-carboxylic acid methyl ester (ITE) is an AhR agonist and has a role in controlling autoimmunity in Treg dependent manner.

As per Abron et al. [85], the activation of the AhR ligand with ITE effectively suppresses inflammatory bowel disease and ameliorates encephalomyelitis symptoms. Additionally, kynurenine and its metabolites are also involved in promoting $FoxP3^+$ immunosuppressive Tregs instead of proinflammatory Th17 cells [86, 87]. In postmenopausal osteoporosis, the imbalance between Tregs and Th17 nexus results in an inflammatory environment. Tryptophan metabolite 5 hydroxy indole acetic acid (5-HIAA) has been observed to prevent bone loss in RA by inducing the Bregs [88]. Supplementing the patient with postbiotics like tryptophan and its metabolites or kynurenine and its metabolites can potentially suppress the inflammation via AhR receptor induction in immune cells.

4.2.4 Phytoestrogens

Phytoestrogens are estrogen-like substances produced from plants that resemble 17-estradiol structurally. Phytoestrogens are classified as isoflavones, stilbene, coumestan, and lignan. Isoflavones are the most studied type of phytoestrogens. Genistein, daidzein, glycitein, formononetin, and biochanin A found in soybeans are the primary isoflavone phytoestrogens [89]. Phytoestrogens are found effective in preventing bone loss due to osteoporosis. Treatment of Ovx rats with resveratrol slowed down the deterioration of trabecular bone [90]. Higher BMD values at the spine and hip regions are seen in postmenopausal women who regularly consume a lot of dietary isoflavones [91]. The trabecular microarchitecture of the proximal tibia in the orchidectomized rat model of male osteoporosis is improved by genistein therapy [92]. Phytoestrogens show immunomodulatory properties due to their ability to block intracellular signaling pathways linked to immunological responses. For instance, genistein can reduce allergic inflammation [89]. Isoflavone extract can lessen the activation of MAPK, NF-κB, and JAK-STAT caused by IL-22, IL-17A, and TNF in healthy human epidermal keratinocytes [93]. Phytoestrogens are also reported to prevent bone loss by modulating the immune system. Treatment with formononetin (formo) and isoformononetin (isoformo) prevented bone loss in ovariectomized mice. In contrast to the Ovx group treated with vehicle, formo/isoformo-treated Ovx mice had lower levels of the pro-osteoclastogenic subset Th17 and B cells. Treatment with formo and isoformo also increased T-regulatory cell differentiation and lowered the expression of Th17 differentiation factors in Ovx mice [94]. Thus, it can be concluded that phytoestrogens can prevent osteoporosis by regulating the immunoporotic axis, but additional research is needed to substantiate this claim.

4.2.5 Biologic therapies

For several systemic inflammatory autoimmune disorders such as RA, inflammatory bowel disease, and psoriasis, biologic therapies targeting crucial elements of the dysregulated immune response have significantly improved patient outcomes and changed treatment paradigms. There are already medicines in the clinic that target specific immune cells like B and T cells or released mediators like proinflammatory cytokines such as TNF, IL-1, IL-6, IL-12, IL-17, and IL-23 [95]. Biologic agents such as etanercept (soluble TNF receptor IgG Fc fusion protein), infliximab, adalimumab, and golimumab (anti-TNF mAbs), certolizumab pegol (pegylated antibody fragment), anakinra (IL-1 receptor antagonist), tocilizumab (anti–IL-6 receptor mAb), ustekinumab (anti–IL-12/IL-23 mAb) and, secukinumab (anti–IL-17A mAb) are permitted for several autoimmune diseases [95]. In the case of RA reduced bone loss is associated with biologic medication therapy. Studies using anti-TNF drugs have shown preservation or growth in the BMD of the spine and the hip, as well as an improved profile of bone markers [96]. The first biologic drug approved for the treatment of osteoporosis was denosumab which increases BMD and reduces fracture risk [97]. Another biologic agent used for osteoporosis treatment is romosozumab [98]. Anti-Dkk-1 monoclonal antibody (PF04840082) is predicted to enhance bone mass and reduce the risk of osteoporotic fractures by encouraging osteoblasts to produce more bone [99]. Thus, these modern antiresorptives or anabolic biologic therapies have the potential to build bone mass quickly to normal levels and decrease fracture rates. Therefore, treatment for osteoporosis can be revolutionized by these more recent medicines [100]. However, more clinical studies are necessary to further prove the effectiveness of biological therapy in preventing osteoporosis while also taking into account their adverse side effects.

5. Conclusion and future prospects

Recent research has demonstrated the critical part the immune system serves in the pathogenesis of osteoporosis. These results open the door for further research in the emerging topic of immunoporosis. Numerous medications used to treat osteoporosis have deadly adverse effects such as nephrotoxicity, ulceration, and BRONJ. A monoclonal antibody targeting RANKL is denosumab. Treatment with denosumab results in a decrease in RANKL-induced osteoclastogenesis. However, many studies have reported that denosumab use causes adverse effects and potentially suppresses the immune system. Many FDA-approved classes of drugs are used for treatment as well, which include selective estrogen receptor modulators (SERMs) and antibodies (the most recent antibody approved was a sclerostin-inhibiting antibody called romosozumab), but side effects with the use of this antibody are also prevalent. Since so many side effects are observed, it is crucial to further investigate the effects of these drugs on the immune system and develop safer therapeutic strategies for targeting the disease. By regulating the immune system, phytotherapy and probiotics, together with their metabolites, have demonstrated extraordinary osteoprotective capabilities and can thus be potential future therapeutic candidates. To confirm their effectiveness in humans, further study is still required because the majority of studies on phytotherapy and probiotics are conducted on mice.

Acknowledgements

VP, TK, AB, LS, SY, and RKS acknowledge the Department of Biotechnology, AIIMS, New Delhi-India for providing infrastructural facilities. AB thanks ICMR, LS thanks UGC, and SY thanks DBT for the research fellowship. Figures are created with the help of Servier Medical Art, provided by Servier, licensed under a Creative Commons Attribution 3.0 unported license (https://smart.servier.com).

Conflicts of interest

The authors declare no conflicts of interest.

Funding

This work was financially supported by projects: DBT(BT/PR41958/MED/97/524/2021), ICMR (61/05/2022-IMM/BMS), and CCRH-AYUSH (614/2022–2023) Govt. of India, and an intramural grant (AC-21) sanctioned to RKS.

Credit authorship contribution statement

RKS contributed to the conceptualization and writing of the manuscript. VP, TK, AB, LS, and SY participated in the writing and editing of the review. RKS suggested and AB created the illustrations.

Author details

Vardhan Pol†, Taranjeet Kaur†, Asha Bhardwaj, Leena Sapra, Sumedha Yadav
and Rupesh K. Srivastava*
Translational Immunology, Osteoimmunology and Immunoporosis Lab, Department
of Biotechnology, All India Institute of Medical Sciences (AIIMS), New Delhi, India

*Address all correspondence to: rupesh_srivastava13@yahoo.co.in

†Authors contributed equally to the manuscript.

References

[1] Cappariello A, Ponzetti M, Rucci N. The "soft" side of the bone: Unveiling its endocrine functions. Hormone Molecular Biology and Clinical Investigation. 2016;**28**(1):5-20

[2] Winkler DG. Osteocyte control of bone formation via sclerostin, a novel BMP antagonist. The EMBO Journal. 2003;**22**(23):6267-6276

[3] Walsh MC, Kim N, Kadono Y, Rho J, Lee SY, Lorenzo J, et al. Osteoimmunology: Interplay between the immune system and bone metabolism. Annual Review of Immunology [Internet]. 2006;**24**:33-63. Available from: http://www.ncbi.nlm.nih.gov/pubmed/16551243

[4] Srivastava RK, Sapra L. The rising era of "Immunoporosis": Role of immune system in the pathophysiology of osteoporosis. Journal of Inflammation Research [Internet]. 2022;**15**:1667-1698. Available from: https://www.dovepress.com/the-rising-era-of-immunoporosis-role-of-immune-system-in-the-pathophys-peer-reviewed-fulltext-article-JIR

[5] Sözen T, Özışık L, Başaran NÇ. An overview and management of osteoporosis. European Journal of Rheumatology [Internet]. 2017;**4**(1):46-56. Available from: http://www.ncbi.nlm.nih.gov/pubmed/28293453

[6] Alnaeeli M, Teng YTA. Dendritic cells differentiate into osteoclasts in bone marrow microenvironment in vivo. Blood. 2009;**113**(1):264-265

[7] Yamaguchi T, Movila A, Kataoka S, Wisitrasameewong W, Ruiz Torruella M, Murakoshi M, et al. Proinflammatory M1 macrophages inhibit RANKL-induced Osteoclastogenesis. Infection and Immunity. 2016;**84**(10):2802-2812

[8] Yang J, Park O, Kim J, Kwon Y, Yun C, Han SH. Modulation of macrophage subtypes by IRF5 determines osteoclastogenic potential. Journal of Cellular Physiology. 2019;**234**(12):23033-23042

[9] Biosse-Duplan M, Baroukh B, Dy M, de Vernejoul MC, Saffar JL. Histamine promotes Osteoclastogenesis through the differential expression of histamine receptors on osteoclasts and osteoblasts. The American Journal of Pathology. 2009;**174**(4):1426-1434

[10] Ginaldi L, De Martinis M, Ciccarelli F, Saitta S, Imbesi S, Mannucci C, et al. Increased levels of interleukin 31 (IL-31) in osteoporosis. BMC Immunology. 2015;**16**(1):60

[11] De Martinis M, Sirufo MM, Suppa M, Ginaldi L. IL-33/IL-31 Axis in osteoporosis. International Journal of Molecular Sciences. 2020;**21**(4):1239

[12] Söderström K, Stein E, Colmenero P, Purath U, Müller-Ladner U, Teixeira de Matos C, et al. Natural killer cells trigger osteoclastogenesis and bone destruction in arthritis. National Academy of Sciences of the United States of America. 2010;**107**(29):13028-13033

[13] Feng S, Madsen SH, Viller NN, Neutzsky-Wulff AV, Geisler C, Karlsson L, et al. Interleukin-15-activated natural killer cells kill autologous osteoclasts via LFA-1, DNAM-1 and TRAIL, and inhibit osteoclast-mediated bone erosion *in vitro*. Immunology. 2015;**145**(3):367-379

[14] Takeda H, Kikuchi T, Soboku K, Okabe I, Mizutani H, Mitani A, et al. Effect of IL-15 and natural killer cells on osteoclasts and osteoblasts

in a mouse coculture. Inflammation. 2014;**37**(3):657-669

[15] Gao Y, Grassi F, Ryan MR, Terauchi M, Page K, Yang X, et al. IFN-γ stimulates osteoclast formation and bone loss in vivo via antigen-driven T cell activation. Journal of Clinical Investigation. 2007;**117**(1):122-132

[16] Tang M, Tian L, Luo G, Yu X. Interferon-gamma-mediated Osteoimmunology. Frontiers in Immunology. 2018;**9**:1508

[17] Place DE, Malireddi RKS, Kim J, Vogel P, Yamamoto M, Kanneganti TD. Osteoclast fusion and bone loss are restrictedbyinterferoninducibleguanylate binding proteins. Nature Communications. 2021;**12**(1):496

[18] Zhang J, Fu Q, Ren Z, Wang Y, Wang C, Shen T, et al. Changes of serum cytokines-related Th1/Th2/Th17 concentration in patients with postmenopausal osteoporosis. Gynecological Endocrinology. 2015;**31**(3):183-190

[19] Mangashetti LS, Khapli SM, Wani MR. IL-4 inhibits bone-resorbing activity of mature osteoclasts by affecting NF-κB and Ca2+ Signaling. The Journal of Immunology. 2005;**175**(2):917-925

[20] Yamada A, Takami M, Kawawa T, Yasuhara R, Zhao B, Mochizuki A, et al. Interleukin-4 inhibition of osteoclast differentiation is stronger than that of interleukin-13 and they are equivalent for induction of osteoprotegerin production from osteoblasts. Immunology. 2007;**120**(4):573-579

[21] Kar S, Gupta R, Malhotra R, Sharma V, Farooque K, Kumar V, et al. Interleukin-9 facilitates Osteoclastogenesis in rheumatoid arthritis. International Journal of Molecular Sciences. 2021;**22**(19):10397

[22] Miyazaki Y, Nakayamada S, Kubo S, Nakano K, Iwata S, Miyagawa I, et al. Th22 cells promote osteoclast differentiation via production of IL-22 in rheumatoid arthritis. Frontiers in Immunology. 2018;**9**:2901

[23] Ma J, Zhu C, Ma B, Tian J, Baidoo SE, Mao C, et al. Increased frequency of circulating follicular helper T cells in patients with rheumatoid arthritis. Clinical & Developmental Immunology. 2012;**2012**:1-7

[24] Niu Q, Chun HZ, Juan WX, Xiong JY, Fei AY, Mei LY, et al. Enhanced IL-6/ phosphorylated STAT3 signaling is related to the imbalance of circulating T follicular helper/T follicular regulatory cells in patients with rheumatoid arthritis. Arthritis Research & Therapy. 2018;**20**(1):200

[25] Kim DH, Park HJ, Park HS, Lee JU, Ko C, Gye MC, et al. Estrogen receptor α in T cells suppresses follicular helper T cell responses and prevents autoimmunity. Experimental & Molecular Medicine. 2019;**51**(4):1-9

[26] Rubinstein MP, Lind NA, Purton JF, Filippou P, Best JA, McGhee PA, et al. IL-7 and IL-15 differentially regulate CD8+ T-cell subsets during contraction of the immune response. Blood. 2008;**112**(9):3704-3712

[27] Ono-Ohmachi A, Yamada S, Uno S, Tamai M, Soga K, Nakamura S, et al. Effector memory CD4+T cells in mesenteric lymph nodes mediate bone loss in food-allergic enteropathy model mice, creating IL-4 dominance. Mucosal Immunology. 2021;**14**(6):1335-1346

[28] Luo C, Wang L, Sun C, Li D. Estrogen enhances the functions of

CD4+CD25+Foxp3+ regulatory T cells that suppress osteoclast differentiation and bone resorption in vitro. Cellular & Molecular Immunology. 2011;**8**(1):50-58

[29] Fischer L, Herkner C, Kitte R, Dohnke S, Riewaldt J, Kretschmer K, et al. Foxp3+ regulatory T cells in bone and hematopoietic homeostasis. Frontiers in Endocrinology (Lausanne). 2019;**10**:578

[30] Kimura A, Kishimoto T. IL-6: Regulator of Treg/Th17 balance. European Journal of Immunology. 2010;**40**(7):1830-1835

[31] Bank I. The role of Gamma Delta T cells in autoimmune rheumatic diseases. Cell. 2020;**9**(2):462

[32] Phalke SP, Chiplunkar SV. Activation status of γδ T cells dictates their effect on osteoclast generation and bone resorption. Bone Reports. 2015;**3**:95-103

[33] Tilkeridis K, Kiziridis G, Ververidis A, Papoutselis M, Kotsianidis I, Kitsikidou G, et al. Immunoporosis: A new role for invariant natural killer T (NKT) cells through overexpression of nuclear factor-κB ligand (RANKL). Medical Science Monitor. 2019;**25**:2151-2158

[34] Onal M, Xiong J, Chen X, Thostenson JD, Almeida M, Manolagas SC, et al. Receptor activator of nuclear factor κB ligand (RANKL) protein expression by B lymphocytes contributes to Ovariectomy-induced bone loss. Journal of Biological Chemistry. 2012;**287**(35):29851-29860

[35] Fujiwara Y, Piemontese M, Liu Y, Thostenson JD, Xiong J, O'Brien CA. RANKL (receptor activator of NFκB ligand) produced by osteocytes is required for the increase in B cells and bone loss caused by estrogen deficiency in mice. Journal of Biological Chemistry. 2016;**291**(48):24838-24850

[36] Sun W, Meednu N, Rosenberg A, Rangel-Moreno J, Wang V, Glanzman J, et al. B cells inhibit bone formation in rheumatoid arthritis by suppressing osteoblast differentiation. Nature Communications. 2018;**9**(1):5127

[37] Sapra L, Bhardwaj A, Kumar Mishra P, Garg B, Verma B, Mishra GC, et al. Regulatory B cells (Bregs) inhibit Osteoclastogenesis and play a potential role in ameliorating Ovariectomy-induced bone loss. Frontiers in Immunology. 2021;**12**:1. Available from: www.frontiersin.org

[38] Yago T, Nanke Y, Kawamoto M, Kobashigawa T, Yamanaka H, Kotake S. IL-35 inhibits human osteoclastogenesis from monocytes induced by receptor-activator of NF-κB ligand. Central European Journal of Immunology. 2018;**43**(2):148-154

[39] Xu Q, Zhan P, Li X, Mo F, Xu H, Liu Y, et al. Bisphosphonate-enoxacin inhibit osteoclast formation and function by abrogating RANKL-induced JNK signalling pathways during osteoporosis treatment. Journal of Cellular and Molecular Medicine. 2021;**25**(21):10126-10139

[40] Kostenuik PJ, Nguyen HQ, McCabe J, Warmington KS, Kurahara C, Sun N, et al. Denosumab, a fully human monoclonal antibody to RANKL, inhibits bone resorption and increases BMD in knock-in mice that express chimeric (murine/human) RANKL. Journal of Bone and Mineral Research. 2009;**24**(2):182-195

[41] Kuo SW, Rimando M, Liu YS, Lee O. Intermittent Administration of Parathyroid Hormone 1-34 enhances Osteogenesis of human mesenchymal

stem cells by regulating protein kinase Cδ. International Journal of Molecular Sciences. 2017;**18**(10):2221

[42] Nada MH, Wang H, Workalemahu G, Tanaka Y, Morita CT. Enhancing adoptive cancer immunotherapy with Vγ2Vδ2 T cells through pulse zoledronate stimulation. Journal for Immunotherapy of Cancer. 2017;**5**(1):9

[43] Liu H, Wang SH, Chen SC, Chen CY, Lo JL, Lin TM. Immune modulation of CD4+CD25+ regulatory T cells by zoledronic acid. BMC Immunology. 2016;**17**(1):45

[44] Tonti E, Jiménez de Oya N, Galliverti G, Moseman EA, Di Lucia P, Amabile A, et al. Bisphosphonates target B cells to enhance humoral immune responses. Cell Reports. 2013;**5**(2):323-330

[45] Yamachika E, Matsui Y, Matsubara M, Matsumura T, Nakata N, Moritani N, et al. The influence of zoledronate and teriparatide on gamma delta T cells in mice. Journal of Dental Sciences. 2017;**12**(4):333-339

[46] Pacifici R. T cells, osteoblasts, and osteocytes: Interacting lineages key for the bone anabolic and catabolic activities of parathyroid hormone. Annals of the New York Academy of Sciences. 2016;**1364**(1):11-24

[47] Mirza FS, Padhi ID, Raisz LG, Lorenzo JA. Serum sclerostin levels negatively correlate with parathyroid hormone levels and free estrogen index in postmenopausal women. The Journal of Clinical Endocrinology and Metabolism. 2010;**95**(4):1991-1997

[48] Bedi B, Li JY, Tawfeek H, Baek KH, Adams J, Vangara SS, et al. Silencing of parathyroid hormone (PTH) receptor 1 in T cells blunts the bone anabolic activity of PTH. Proceedings of the National Academy of Sciences. 2012;**109**(12):E725-E733

[49] Terauchi M, Li JY, Bedi B, Baek KH, Tawfeek H, Galley S, et al. T lymphocytes amplify the anabolic activity of parathyroid hormone through Wnt10b signaling. Cell Metabolism. 2009;**10**(3):229-240

[50] Yu M, D'Amelio P, Tyagi AM, Vaccaro C, Li J, Hsu E, et al. Regulatory T cells are expanded by teriparatide treatment in humans and mediate intermittent PTH-induced bone anabolism in mice. EMBO Reports. 2018;**19**(1):156-171

[51] Panaroni C, Fulzele K, Saini V, Chubb R, Pajevic PD, Wu JY. PTH signaling in osteoprogenitors is essential for B-lymphocyte differentiation and mobilization. Journal of Bone and Mineral Research. 2015;**30**(12):2273-2286

[52] Wensel TM, Iranikhah MM, Wilborn TW. Effects of denosumab on bone mineral density and bone turnover in postmenopausal women. Pharmacotherapy. 2011;**31**(5):510-523

[53] Rossini M, Viapiana O, Adami S, Idolazzi L, Ghellere F, Tripi G, et al. Effects of denosumab on peripheral lymphocyte subpopulations. Endocrine. 2016;**53**(3):857-859

[54] Fabre S, Funck-Brentano T, Cohen-Solal M. Anti-Sclerostin antibodies in osteoporosis and other bone diseases. Journal of Clinical Medicine. 2020;**9**(11):3439

[55] Cosman F, Crittenden DB, Adachi JD, Binkley N, Czerwinski E, Ferrari S, et al. Romosozumab treatment in postmenopausal women with osteoporosis. New England Journal of Medicine. 2016;**375**(16):1532-1543

[56] Geusens P, Oates M, Miyauchi A, Adachi JD, Lazaretti-Castro M, Ebeling PR, et al. The effect of 1 year of romosozumab on the incidence of clinical vertebral fractures in postmenopausal women with osteoporosis: Results from the FRAME study. JBMR Plus. 2019;**3**(10):e10211

[57] Lim SY, Bolster MB. Clinical utility of romosozumab in the management of Osteoporosis: Focus on patient selection and perspectives. International Journal of Women's Health. 2022;**14**:1733-1747

[58] Pennypacker B, Shea M, Liu Q, Masarachia P, Saftig P, Rodan S, et al. Bone density, strength, and formation in adult cathepsin K (−/−) mice. Bone. 2009;**44**(2):199-207

[59] Kiviranta R, Morko J, Uusitalo H, Aro HT, Vuorio E, Rantakokko J. Accelerated turnover of metaphyseal trabecular bone in mice overexpressing cathepsin K. Journal of Bone and Mineral Research. 2001;**16**(8):1444-1452

[60] Duong LT, Leung AT, Langdahl B. Cathepsin K inhibition: A new mechanism for the treatment of osteoporosis. Calcified Tissue International. 2016;**98**(4):381-397

[61] Yates J, Barrett-Connor E, Barlas S, Chen YT, Miller PD, Siris ES. Rapid loss of hip fracture protection after estrogen cessation: Evidence from the National osteoporosis risk assessment. Obstetrics & Gynecology. 2004;**103**(3):440-446

[62] Mehta J, Kling JM, Manson JE. Risks, benefits, and treatment modalities of menopausal hormone therapy: Current concepts. Frontiers in Endocrinology (Lausanne). 2021;**12**:564781

[63] Gambacciani M, Levancini M. Featured editorial hormone replacement therapy and the prevention of postmenopausal osteoporosis. Menopausal Review. 2014;**4**:213-220

[64] Sapra L, Shokeen N, Porwal K, Saini C, Bhardwaj A, Mathew M, et al. Bifidobacterium longum ameliorates ovariectomy-induced bone loss via enhancing anti-osteoclastogenic and immunomodulatory potential of regulatory B cells (Bregs). Frontiers in Immunology. 2022;**13**:875788

[65] Azam Z, Sapra L, Baghel K, Sinha N, Gupta RK, Soni V, et al. Cissus quadrangularis (Hadjod) inhibits RANKL-induced osteoclastogenesis and augments bone health in an estrogen-deficient preclinical model of osteoporosis via modulating the host osteoimmune system. Cell. 2023;**12**(2):216

[66] Chen X, Zhi X, Yin Z, Li X, Qin L, Qiu Z, et al. 18β-glycyrrhetinic acid inhibits osteoclastogenesis in vivo and in vitro by blocking RANKL-mediated RANK–TRAF6 interactions and NF-κB and MAPK signaling pathways. Frontiers in Pharmacology. 2018;**9**:647

[67] Yang C, Zhu K, Yuan X, Zhang X, Qian Y, Cheng T. Curcumin has immunomodulatory effects on RANKL-stimulated osteoclastogenesis in vitro and titanium nanoparticle-induced bone loss in vivo. Journal of Cellular and Molecular Medicine. 2020;**24**(2):1553-1567

[68] Chen H, Fang C, Zhi X, Song S, Gu Y, Chen X, et al. Neobavaisoflavone inhibits osteoclastogenesis through blocking RANKL signalling-mediated TRAF6 and c-Src recruitment and NF-κB, MAPK and Akt pathways. Journal of Cellular and Molecular Medicine. 2020;**24**(16):9067-9084

[69] Fu L, Pan F, Jiao Y. Crocin inhibits RANKL-induced osteoclast formation

and bone resorption by suppressing NF-κB signaling pathway activation. Immunobiology. 2017;**222**(4):597-603

[70] Shi L, Zhao S, Chen Q, Wu Y, Zhang J, Li N. Crocin inhibits RANKL-induced osteoclastogenesis by regulating JNK and NF-κB signaling pathways. Molecular Medicine Reports. 2018;**17**(6):7947-7951

[71] Azam Z, Sapra L, Bhardwaj A, Yadav S, Mishra PK, Shukla P, et al. Crocin attenuates osteoclastogenesis and enhances bone health by skewing the immunoporotic "Treg-Th17" cell axis in post-menopausal osteoporotic mice model. Phytomedicine Plus. 2022;**2**(3):100302

[72] McCabe LR, Irwin R, Schaefer L, Britton RA. Probiotic use decreases intestinal inflammation and increases bone density in healthy male but not female mice. Journal of Cellular Physiology. 2013;**228**(8):1793-1798

[73] Srivastava RK, Dar HY, Mishra PK. Immunoporosis: Immunology of osteoporosis—Role of T cells. Frontiers in Immunology. 2018;**9**:657

[74] Sapra L, Azam Z, Rani L, Saini C, Bhardwaj A, Shokeen N, et al. "Immunoporosis": Immunology of osteoporosis. Proceedings of the National Academy of Sciences, India Section B: Biological Sciences [Internet]. 2021;**91**(3):511-519. Available from: https://link.springer.com/10.1007/s40011-021-01238-x

[75] Sapra L, Dar HY, Bhardwaj A, Pandey A, Kumari S, Azam Z, et al. Lactobacillus rhamnosus attenuates bone loss and maintains bone health by skewing Treg-Th17 cell balance in Ovx mice. Scientific Reports [Internet]. 2021;**11**(1):1807. DOI: 10.1038/s41598-020-80536-2

[76] Dar HY, Pal S, Shukla P, Mishra PK, Tomar GB, Chattopadhyay N, et al. Bacillus clausii inhibits bone loss by skewing Treg-Th17 cell equilibrium in postmenopausal osteoporotic mice model. Nutrition [Internet]. 2018;**54**:118-128. Available from: http://www.ncbi.nlm.nih.gov/pubmed/29793054

[77] Dar HY, Shukla P, Mishra PK, Anupam R, Mondal RK, Tomar GB, et al. Lactobacillus acidophilus inhibits bone loss and increases bone heterogeneity in osteoporotic mice via modulating Treg-Th17 cell balance. Bone Reports [Internet]. 2018;**8**:46-56. Available from: http://www.ncbi.nlm.nih.gov/pubmed/29955622

[78] Mariño E, Richards JL, McLeod KH, Stanley D, Yap YA, Knight J, et al. Gut microbial metabolites limit the frequency of autoimmune T cells and protect against type 1 diabetes. Nature Immunology. 2017;**18**(5):552-562

[79] Lucas S, Omata Y, Hofmann J, Böttcher M, Iljazovic A, Sarter K, et al. Short-chain fatty acids regulate systemic bone mass and protect from pathological bone loss. Nature Communications [Internet]. 2018;**9**(1):55. Available from: http://www.nature.com/articles/s41467-017-02490-4

[80] Hang S, Paik D, Yao L, Kim E, Trinath J, Lu J, et al. Bile acid metabolites control TH17 and Treg cell differentiation. Nature. 2019;**576**(7785):143-148

[81] Li W, Hang S, Fang Y, Bae S, Zhang Y, Zhang M, et al. A bacterial bile acid metabolite modulates Treg activity through the nuclear hormone receptor NR4A1. Cell Host & Microbe. 2021;**29**(9):1366-1377.e9

[82] Dubreuil M, Ruiz-Gaspà S, Guañabens N, Peris P, Álvarez L,

Monegal A, et al. Ursodeoxycholic acid increases differentiation and mineralization and neutralizes the damaging effects of bilirubin on osteoblastic cells. Liver International. 2013;**33**(7):1029-1038

[83] Li Z, Huang J, Wang F, Li W, Wu X, Zhao C, et al. Dual targeting of bile acid receptor-1 (TGR5) and Farnesoid X receptor (FXR) prevents estrogen-dependent bone loss in mice. Journal of Bone and Mineral Research. 2018;**34**(4):765-776; jbmr.3652

[84] Gandhi R, Kumar D, Burns EJ, Nadeau M, Dake B, Laroni A, et al. Activation of the aryl hydrocarbon receptor induces human type 1 regulatory T cell–like and Foxp3+ regulatory T cells. Nature Immunology. 2010;**11**(9):846-853

[85] Abron JD, Singh NP, Mishra MK, Price RL, Nagarkatti M, Nagarkatti PS, et al. An endogenous aryl hydrocarbon receptor ligand, ITE, induces regulatory T cells and ameliorates experimental colitis. American Journal of Physiology-Gastrointestinal and Liver Physiology. 2018;**315**(2):G220-G230

[86] Bessede A, Gargaro M, Pallotta MT, Matino D, Servillo G, Brunacci C, et al. Aryl hydrocarbon receptor control of a disease tolerance defence pathway. Nature. 2014;**511**(7508):184-190

[87] Masuda K, Kimura A, Hanieh H, Nguyen NT, Nakahama T, Chinen I, et al. Aryl hydrocarbon receptor negatively regulates LPS-induced IL-6 production through suppression of histamine production in macrophages. International Immunology. 2011;**23**(10):637-645

[88] Rosser EC, Piper CJM, Matei DE, Blair PA, Rendeiro AF, Orford M, et al. Microbiota-derived metabolites suppress arthritis by amplifying aryl-hydrocarbon receptor activation in regulatory B cells. Cell Metabolism [Internet]. 2020;**31**(4):837-851.e10. Available from: https://linkinghub.elsevier.com/retrieve/pii/S1550413120301182

[89] Desmawati D, Sulastri D. Phytoestrogens and their health effect. Open Access Macedonian Journal of Medical Sciences. 2019;**7**(3):495-499

[90] Zaychenko G, Belenichev I, Hnatiuk V, Doroshenko A, Sinitsyna O, Sulaieva O, et al. Protective effect of vaginal resveratrol administration on joint tissues in ovariectomized rats: Targeting mTOR and caspase 3. Biomedicine & Pharmacotherapy. 2023;**165**:115176

[91] Mei J, Yeung SSC, Kung AWC. High dietary phytoestrogen intake is associated with higher bone mineral density in postmenopausal but not premenopausal women. The Journal of Clinical Endocrinology and Metabolism. 2001;**86**(11):5217-5221

[92] Filipović B, Šošić-Jurjević B, Ajdžanović V, Živanović J, Manojlović-Stojanoski M, Nestorović N, et al. The phytoestrogen genistein prevents trabecular bone loss and affects thyroid follicular cells in a male rat model of osteoporosis. Journal of Anatomy. 2018;**233**(2):204-212

[93] Li HJ, Wu NL, Lee GA, Hung CF. The therapeutic potential and molecular mechanism of Isoflavone extract against psoriasis. Scientific Reports. 2018;**8**(1):6335

[94] Mansoori MN, Tyagi AM, Shukla P, Srivastava K, Dev K, Chillara R, et al. Methoxyisoflavones formononetin and isoformononetin inhibit the differentiation of Th17 cells and B-cell lymphopoesis to promote osteogenesis in

estrogen-deficient bone loss conditions. Menopause. 2016;**23**(5):565-576

[95] Her M, Kavanaugh A. Alterations in immune function with biologic therapies for autoimmune disease. Journal of Allergy and Clinical Immunology. 2016;**137**(1):19-27

[96] Zerbini CAF, Clark P, Mendez-Sanchez L, Pereira RMR, Messina OD, Uña CR, et al. Biologic therapies and bone loss in rheumatoid arthritis. Osteoporosis International. 2017;**28**(2):429-446

[97] Tu KN, Lie JD, Wan CKV, Cameron M, Austel AG, Nguyen JK, et al. Osteoporosis: A review of treatment options. P T. 2018;**43**(2):92-104

[98] Rosen CJ, Ingelfinger JR. Building better bones with biologics — A new approach to osteoporosis? New England Journal of Medicine. 2016;**375**(16):1583-1584

[99] Betts AM, Clark TH, Yang J, Treadway JL, Li M, Giovanelli MA, et al. The application of target information and preclinical pharmacokinetic/ pharmacodynamic modeling in predicting clinical doses of a Dickkopf-1 antibody for osteoporosis. The Journal of Pharmacology and Experimental Therapeutics. 2010;**333**(1):2-13

[100] Tella SH, Gallagher JC. Biological agents in management of osteoporosis. European Journal of Clinical Pharmacology. 2014;**70**(11):1291-1301

Chapter 3

Immunology and Osteoporosis: A New Frontier in Treatment

Riya Mukherjee, Chung-Ming Chang and Ramendra Pati Pandey

Abstract

Osteoporosis, a chronic bone disease, alters both the microstructure and macrostructure of bones, endangering bone strength and increasing the susceptibility to fragility fractures. Its consequences on the aging population raise important sociological, healthcare, and economic issues. The relationship between the immune system and osteoporosis can be understood by carefully examining a wide range of immune cells, related cytokines, and their functions. Long-term inflammation, immune cell production of RANKL, and autoimmune illnesses like systemic lupus erythematosus and rheumatoid arthritis all affect bone loss. An overview of the cycle of bone remodeling and the pathophysiology of osteoporosis are covered in this chapter. Important features of osteoporosis for diagnostic purposes are covered, including the formation and resorption markers, potential immunological markers for osteoporosis diagnosis, and new bone metabolic biomarkers. This chapter focuses solely on the roles of innate and adaptive immune cells. It also highlights novel therapeutic strategies that target specific immune pathways and show promise in the management of these challenging bone disorders. As research advances, these findings may pave the way for more specialized and efficient treatments, ultimately enhancing the quality of life for osteoporosis patients.

Keywords: osteoporosis, immune system, immunoporosis, biomarkers, immunotherapy

1. Introduction

Osteoporosis is a chronic bone disease that weakens bone mass and raises the risk of fragility fractures by affecting both the microstructure and macrostructure of bone. The bones typically affected are those in the hip and spine. The condition's deterioration with age is a significant public health issue with clear social, health, and financial consequences. The most significant way that it lowers people's quality of life is by causing pain and functional restrictions. People over 50 are typically more likely to develop osteoporosis. Women (16.5%) and males (5.1%) both had significantly higher prevalence rates. By 2025, 121.3 million people would be estimated to have osteoporosis and low bone mass [1]. Prior to the development of osteoporosis, there are no warning indications or symptoms. It silently depletes bone mass up until a fragility fracture occurs. Osteoporosis risk factors include malnutrition-related deficiencies in calcium and vitamin D, sedentary habits or insufficient exercise, and use of tobacco and alcohol. Other secondary causes have been discovered, such as celiac disease, chronic renal failure, monoclonal gammopathy of unknown origin, renal tubular acidosis, and diabetic mellitus [2].

Osteoporosis is diagnosed by dual-energy X-ray absorptiometry (DEXA), which gauges bone mineral density. The WHO suggests utilizing the fracture risk prediction (FRAX) tool to measure the frequency of osteoporotic fractures [3]. The sole foundation for treatment is the pathophysiology of osteoporosis, which is studied at various stages of disease progression. Healthy bone has dynamic and balanced production and resorption. Therefore, drugs that inhibit resorption and promote bone formation are used to treat osteoporosis. To find new target factors for osteoporosis treatment, research approaches now prioritize examining the genomes, proteomes, epigenomes, and metabolomes of human samples. One of the recommended treatments for osteoporosis is prevention. Bone tissue ossifies, grows, and undergoes changes. These processes are necessary for the consistency or strength of the bone, and to maintain them, certain nutrition and exercises are essential. By maintaining a balanced diet that includes the nutrients required for bone synthesis, growth, and maintenance, osteoporosis can be prevented. Recent research in this area has shown that some of the medicines used to treat osteoporosis, such as bisphosphonates, estrogens, mesenchymal stem cell therapies, and vitamin D supplementation, can alter immunological mediators. The term "immunoporosis" emphasizes how immune cells contribute to osteoporosis. One of the main initiators of many bone illnesses is inflammation. Latest study has shown that osteoblast pyroptosis, or inflammatory cell death, is essential for osteoporosis. Acute inflammatory illnesses are brought on by a variety of signals, including exogenous signals PAMPS (Pathogen Associated Molecular Patterns) and endogenous signals DAMPS (Death Associated Molecular Patterns), which cause inflammation in the body and rapidly assault the immune system. In this chapter, the overview of pathophysiology of osteoporosis, immunological markers, and immunotherapy for osteoporosis are described. This chapter will provide in-depth information about the immunology of osteoporosis as a new treatment approach.

2. Pathophysiology and alterations of bone structure

Bone is a distinctive, multifaceted connective tissue that contains both organic and inorganic elements. Bone has constant turnover throughout adulthood. As a result, bone tissue is renewed, keeping the skeleton's biomechanical characteristics. A wide variety of non-collagenous proteins as well as collagenous proteins make up the osteoid, organic bone matrix. The numerous non-collagenous proteins control the deposition, mineralization, and turnover of bones, among other aspects of bone metabolism. The inorganic component, which makes up between 50 and 70 percent of the total bone mass, is mostly composed of calcium and phosphorus in the form of hydroxyapatite and gives the bone its mechanical firmness. Osteocytes, osteoblasts, and osteoclasts make up most of the cells that make up bone's cellular structure. Osteocytes play a mechano-sensory role in bone formation and are in the matrix's lacunae. While osteoclasts enzymatically resorb bone, osteoblasts produce osteoid [4].

A delicate balance between the actions of osteoclasts and osteoblasts is required for bone remodeling to maintain skeletal structure, repair microdamage, and

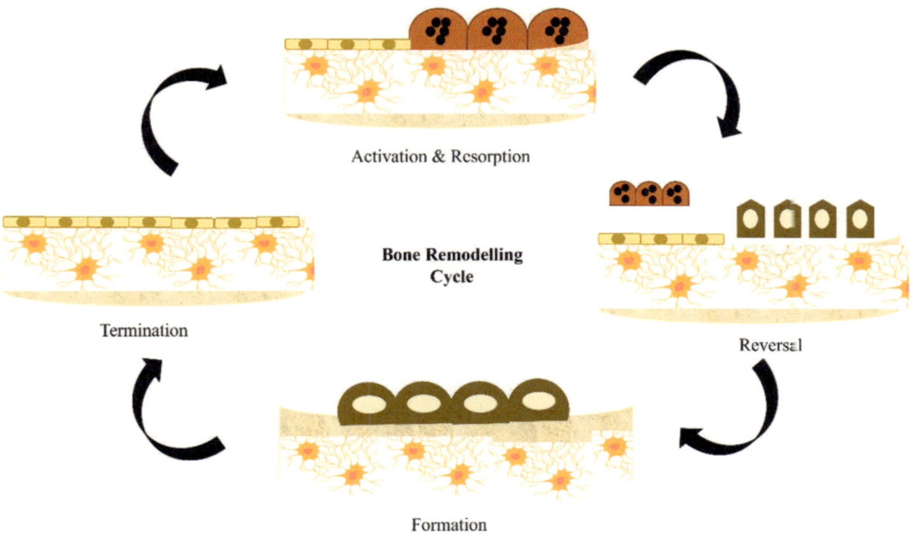

Figure 1.
The phases of bone remodeling cycle.

maintain serum calcium and phosphate homeostasis. A specific sequence of cellular activities taking place at a specific location on the trabecular bone surfaces or in cortical bone make up the process of bone remodeling. The five steps of the remodeling cycle on the surface of the resting bone are activation, resorption, reversal, formation, and termination (**Figure 1**). The first stage is activation, which causes the lining cells to retract back from the surface of the bone. Osteoclast precursors multiply and develop into adult osteoclasts in the bone marrow. Osteoclasts destroy the old bone by secreting hydrogen ions and lysosomal enzymes from beneath the cell, which causes acidification and proteolysis. This particular area of the bone surface is where these active osteoclasts are drawn to. The nuclear factor NF- kB ligand amino acid peptide receptor activator, which binds to the kB ligand receptor on osteoclast precursors and may drive development into multinucleated osteoclasts, is expressed by osteoocytes. The expression of M-CSF (macrophage colony-stimulating factor) by osteoblasts promotes the survival and growth of osteoclast precursors. Osteoblasts create matrix metalloproteinase to degrade our calcified osteoid and expose adhesion sites for osteoclast attachment. Osteoblasts create chemokines to entice potential osteoclast precursors [4].

The second step is the phase of bone resorption by osteoclasts which will excavate an erosion cavity. Osteoprotegerin (OPG) prevents the interaction between kB-kB, which lowers resorption by preventing osteoclast development and raising their death [4]. The next stage, known as the reversal phase, involves the preparation of the bone lacuna by mononuclear cells. The critical connection of osteoclastic and osteoblastic activity found at remodeling sites is caused by the reversal phase, which starts with osteoclastic signaling [5]. They promote osteoblast differentiation and proliferative growth. To entirely replace the tunnel of resorbed bone, osteoblasts deposit un-mineralized osteoid, which results in a limited net change in bone volume during remodeling. As osteoid gradually mineralizes by incorporating hydroxyapatite, bone formation is finished. The remodeling cycle is complete when the tunnel of resorbed bone has been completely restored [6].

3. Osteoimmunology

Osteoporosis is traditionally thought of as the result of an estrogen-driven dysregulation of the bone remodeling process. However, new developments in the field have now firmly proven the immune system's crucial role in regulating inflammatory bone loss in osteoporotic disorders, or "Immunoporosis," i.e., osteoporosis. We emphasize the distinct functions of diverse innate and adaptive immune cells and their plasticity, and we uncover fresh therapeutic prospects for clinical interventions as well as their applicability in various pathological states of the bone, including osteoporosis (**Figures 2** and **3**).

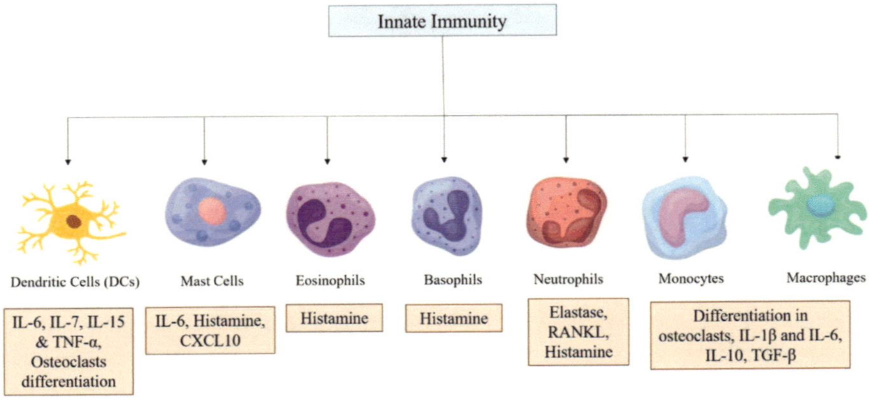

Figure 2.
Schematic diagram representing the role of immune cells and their cytokines in the pathophysiology of osteoporosis.

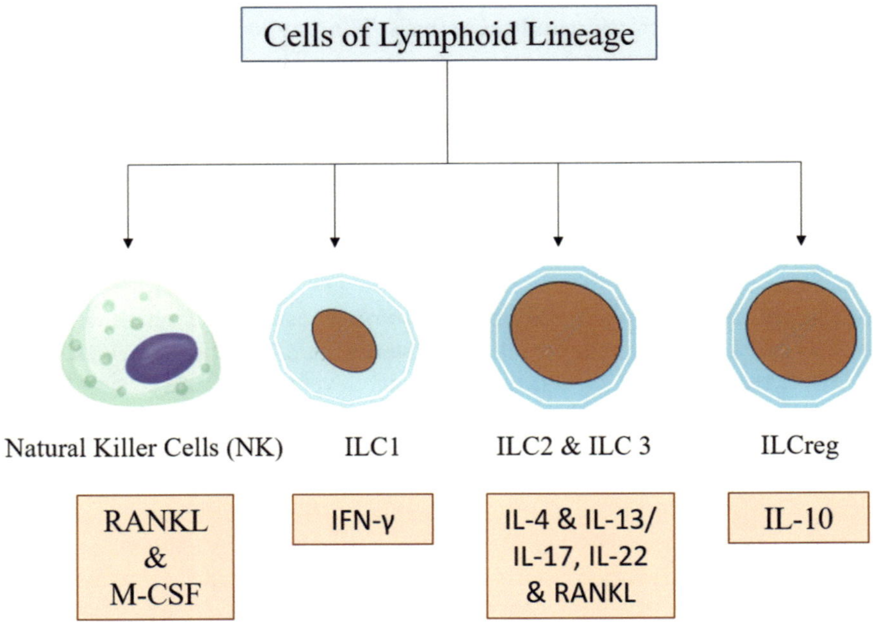

Figure 3.
Schematic diagram representing the role of lymphoid lineage and their cytokines in the pathophysiology of osteoporosis.

3.1 Role of innate immune cells in osteoporosis

The term "myeloid lineage" refers to the type of bone marrow cell development pathway that gives rise to different types of immune cells (**Table 1**). As the first line of defense against any invasive pathogens within the host, innate immune cells are also the main makers of pro-inflammatory mediators, which serve as triggers for the emergence of a number of bone diseases, including osteoporosis. According to a study, Macrophages, OC's, and DC's are all clinically significant cells because they all originate from the same progenitor [9]. In addition to these cells, the production of numerous inflammatory mediators by granulocytes, innate lymphoid cells (ILCs), and natural killer (NK) cells further promotes the development of osteoporosis. The body's fight against illnesses and infections depends heavily on these cells. TNF-α, IL-1β, ROS, and IFN-γ are a few of the main pro-inflammatory mediators that are released by innate immune cells (**Table 2**) [18].

Cell type	Physiological role	Function
Macrophage	Inflammation, tissue repair	M1 macrophage promotes bone rescrption, M2 macrophage majorly promotes bone formation by stimulating differentiation of precursor cells into mature osteoblasts [7, 8].
Monocyte	Inflammation	Serves as precursor to osteoclasts, macrophages and DCs [9].
Dendritic Cells (DCs)	Inflammation, antigen presentation	Can transdifferentiate to osteoclasts in the inflammatory milieu [10].
Neutrophils	Inflammation, Phagosytosis	Promotes bone resorption by increased expression of mRANKL [11].
Mast Cells	Allergic Response, Inflammation	Triggers osteoclastogenesis by producing pro-inflammatory mediators [12].
NK Cells	Cellular cytotoxicity, AdCC, Inflammation	Promotes osteoclastogenesis by producing RANKL and MCSF [13].

Table 1.
Innate immune cell types and their role in osteoimmunology.

Pro-inflammatory cytokines	Cellular sources	Functions
TNF-α	T-cells, NK cells, B cells, Neutrophils, Monocytes, Macrophages.	promotes RANK expression on macrophages and stromal cell production of RANKL, limiting osteoblast development, proliferation, and activity [14].
IFN- γ	T-cells, NK cells, B-cells, Neutrophils, Monocytes, Macrophages.	T-cell activation and osteoclast fusion [15].
IL-6	Osteoblasts, Osteoclasts, Dendritic cells, Macrophages.	Osteoclast activation and migration are mediated by RANK-L [16, 17].

Table 2.
Role of pro-inflammatory cytokines in osteoimmunology.

3.1.1 Macrophages

The most powerful inflammatory cells, macrophages, serve as the main sentinel cells. They exist in the tissues and are capable of quickly detecting pathogen infection caused by bacteria, viruses, parasites, etc. They also operate as a host system's first line of defense. They have the capacity to trigger inflammatory reactions as well as phagocytosis. This capability results from the presence of a wide variety of pattern recognition receptors (PRRs), including scavenger receptors (SRs), toll receptors (TLRs), nod-like receptors (NLRs), etc. Bone marrow macrophages (BMMs), OCs, and osteal macrophages are among the several macrophage populations found in the bone [7]. Osteal macrophages aid in the effective mineralization of osteoblasts and the production of bone. Bone mineral density (BMD) is shown to decline in the presence of osteal macrophages. In addition to causing inflammation, macrophages support tissue homeostasis and assist in tissue healing after injury [8, 9]. They have a high degree of flexibility to support these functions and can switch between an M1 and M2 phenotype depending on the surroundings. Both M1 and M2 are alternatively activated macrophages; M1 is a classically activated macrophage. Bone remodeling processes are driven by macrophage polarization. Anti-inflammatory cytokines like IL-4 and IL-13 can induce M2 polarization, which is typically linked to bone catabolic and anabolic activities, whereas pro-inflammatory cytokines like TNF-α and IL-6 can stimulate M1 polarization [19].

M2 macrophages have been implicated in osteogenesis in numerous studies. An osteoclast's precursor is the M1 macrophage. By generating pro-inflammatory cytokines including TNF-α, IL-1β, and IL-6, which can promote osteoclastogenesis and bone resorption, macrophages are widely acknowledged to play a crucial part in the pathogenesis of the inflammatory disease rheumatoid arthritis (RA). In osteoarthritis (OA) and peri-implant osteolysis, macrophages were also seen to contribute in similar ways [9].

3.1.2 Monocytes

Monocytes make up 10% of all leukocytes in humans and 2–4% in mice. Similar to macrophages, different subsets of monocytes exist, and each has particular traits and functions [20]. Monocytes can participate directly in the inflammatory process in addition to acting only as precursors. As a result of serving as precursors for osteoclasts and producing cytokines, circulating monocytes have a big impact on bone remodeling. Monocytes may also play a significant role in bone issues, as evidenced by the fact that intermediate monocytes take the initiative to transform into high bone-absorbing osteoclasts and may result in bone degeneration [9].

3.1.3 Dendritic cells

Antigen-presenting cells (APCs) with the capacity to elicit an adaptive immune response make up the majority of dendritic cells (DC). The process of bone resorption, osteoclastogenesis, which is mediated by inflammation, can be aided by DCs. T-cells that have been stimulated by DCs can also release cytokines and soluble substances that promote bone remodeling. Furthermore, DCs and T-cells can work together directly to create aggregates that are involved in bone diseases. TGF-, a strong anti-osteoporotic molecule, is known to be produced by DCs. This suggests an alternative function for DCs in osteoporosis [21].

3.1.4 Neutrophils

Additionally, neutrophils can cause osteoporosis by secreting substances that promote osteoclastogenesis and increased bone resorption. Neutrophils have the ability to make chemokines and draw in osteoporotic cells like Th17. Neutrophils can increase bone loss, but they can prevent it by keeping the body's homeostasis in check [22].

3.1.5 Eosinophils & mast cells

Eosinophils are responsible for allergic reactions and the production of pro-inflammatory cytokines including IL-31, which plays a role in controlling transcription factors and cytokines linked to osteoporosis. Mast cells play a role in both physiological processes and the pathophysiology of many diseases, including problems with the bones. They release inflammatory mediators that control bone homeostasis and trigger osteoclastogenesis, such as histamine and TNF-α [9].

3.1.6 Natural killer cells

Natural killer cells (NK) are crucial for maintaining homesostasis and immunoregulation because they regulate the activity of T-cells. They aid in the development of inflammatory illnesses by triggering inflammatory processes and cytotoxicity. NK cells have been observed in synovial regions that are inflamed at an early stage of RA, according to certain publications. Both M-CSF and factor-kB ligand (RANKL), which are potent osteoclastogenesis activators, are produced by these NK cells [13].

3.1.7 Innate lymphoid cells (ILCs)

A boom in study led to the discovery of the innate lymphoid cells (ILCs), a newly emerging component of the innate immune system. ILCs were categorized into three groups; Group 1, Group 2, and Group 3 ILCs. ILC1 and NK cells are in Group 1. T-box transcription factor (T-bet) and IFN- cytokine are essential for the growth and operation of these cells. ILC2 is a member of Group 2 and secretes IL-4, IL-5, IL-9, and IL-13 cytokines. ILC2 depends on the transcription factors GATA binding protein-3 (GATA-3) and retinoic acid receptor-related orphan receptor alpha (ROR) for its development. ILC3 and lymphoid tissue inducer cells (LTi), which depend on the transcription factor RORt for their growth and release the cytokines IL-17 and IL-22, are members of group 3. The expression of either the CC chemokine receptor-6 (CCR-6) or the natural cytotoxicity receptor (NCR), which consists of NKp30, NKp44, and NKp46, further categorizes ILC3s into subsets. ILCs are a new class of lymphocytes that mimic the appearance and capabilities of T helper cells. ILC1, ILC2, and ILC3 are analogous to the Th1, Th2, and Th17 CD4+ T helper cells of the adaptive immune system, respectively, in terms of origin and function. ILCs have been identified to have a role in tissue remodeling, defense against infections, and tissue homeostasis. They are primarily concentrated at barrier surfaces. The pathophysiology of inflammatory and autoimmune disorders such multiple sclerosis (MS), inflammatory bowel disease (IBD), rheumatoid arthritis (RA), and anti-neutrophil cytoplasmic antibody (ANCA) linked vasculitis has been linked to dysregulation in the activation of ILCs, according to several studies [23, 24].

3.1.8 ILC1

Similar to Th1, ILC1 relies on T-bet for development and generates large amounts of the hallmark cytokine IFN- to defend against inflammatory diseases and intracellular infections. ILC1s activate conventional macrophages in response to the intracellular pathogen by using IFN-. ILC1 cells, which share similarities with Th1-cell type, have the potential to reduce bone loss in a mouse model of osteoporosis by producing IFN-. ILCs have been found to release RANKL, which has the potential to improve the differentiation of OCs [24].

3.1.9 ILC2 & ILC3

ILC2s can be considered as the innate equivalent of Th2 cells. According to a study, ILC2s reduced osteoclastogenesis both in vivo and in vitro by releasing IL-4 and IL-13 cytokines. The generation of IL-4/IL-13 cytokines and STAT6 activation in OCs progenitors were linked to ILC2's anti-osteoclastogenic and anti-osteoporotic properties. The innate counterparts of Th17 cells are ILC3s. ILC3s are dependent on the production of reactive oxygen species and a metabolic pathway that integrates glycolysis and mitochondrial lipid oxidation [24].

3.1.10 ILCregs

ILCregs are a type of innate lymphoid cells that have a distinct genetic identity from other ILC subpopulations and regulatory T cells. They are present in the gastrointestinal tracts of both humans and mice and are responsible for regulating immune responses. These cells can reduce the activation of ILC1 and ILC3 by secreting IL-10, which supports the resolution of intestinal inflammation. The discovery of ILCregs' immunosuppressive activities through the secretion of IL-10 could lead to new research avenues and suggest their potential role in controlling osteoporosis [25].

3.2 Role of adaptive immune cells in osteoporosis

The adaptive immune system is crucial in preventing reinfection from pathogens by providing various resistance strategies and memory responses. B and T cells are significant elements of the adaptive immune system, and they have the potential to impact bone health in osteoporosis. In this section, we will delve into the role of these lymphocytes in osteoporosis.

3.2.1 T cells

The T cells of the adaptive immune system play a crucial role in maintaining bone health. When T cells are at rest, they can prevent osteoclasts (OCs) from breaking down bone. However, when activated, they can increase bone resorption by promoting the production of OCs through the production of RANKL. Studies have shown that interferon-gamma (IFN-γ) has a negative correlation with T cell activation and the process of bone resorption. IFN-γ interferes with RANKL-RANK signaling, leading to the degradation of the RANK adaptor protein (TRAF6) and inhibiting osteoclastogenesis [26].

3.2.2 Tregs/Th17 cells

The balance between regulatory T cells (Tregs) and inflammatory T cells (Th17) is crucial for maintaining immunological homeostasis, and research into these cells has experienced an unprecedented boom. Pathogenesis of bone-related illnesses, including osteoporosis, is heavily influenced by an imbalance between these immune cells. Th17 cells are T effector cells, but pTregs and tTregs, which are generated from the thymus, are both members of the regulatory cell lineage. According to a study, pTregs are locally involved in regulating effector activities of T cells at the site of inflammation, whereas tTregs are involved in the maintenance of immunological homeostasis and broad-spectrum autoimmune disorders [24].

3.2.3 Memory T cells

After the initial antigenic exposure, memory T cells are produced, and they are essential for maintaining robust immune responses against these antigens. BM is where memory T cells often reside since it offers a suitable environment for their self-renewal. DCs have been seen to live longer and express more IL-7 and IL-15 cytokines in estrogen-deficient environments. Together, these cytokines cause memory T cells to produce IL-17A and TNF- without the need for an antigen [27].

3.2.4 B cells & regulatory B cells (Bregs)

The potential of B cells in osteo-immunological regulation is being highlighted by new research, which is further validated by the physiological and anatomical coexistence of B cells and bone cells in BM. According to a paper, RANKL not only improves OC development but also boosts the amount of B cells, which serve as an additional OC supporting cell. Numerous studies have shown that B cells have "non-humoral" functions, or immunomodulatory qualities that are independent of secreting antibodies [24].

The immunosuppressive subset of B cells in the B cell lineage known as regulatory B cells (Bregs) is known to inhibit inflammation in a variety of autoimmune and inflammatory disorders. Bregs have been found to inhibit the progression of arthritis by releasing the cytokine IL-10 in the arthritic model. The subpopulation of Bregs, CD19 + CD1dhiCD5+, which is highly enriched for IL-10, has characteristics that can inhibit osteoclastogenesis. In bone fracture patients, the frequencies of IL-10-producing Bregs (IgM + CD27+) were significantly increased during the early healing state (6 weeks after surgery), indicating the role of Bregs in mediating the fracture healing process [24].

4. Immune dysfunction and osteoporosis

Immune cells and inflammatory chemicals are essential for bone remodeling, and immune system dysregulation can cause bone loss and the onset of osteoporosis.

i. *Inflammatory cytokines*: Chronic inflammation, which is characterized by increased production of pro-inflammatory cytokines like interleukin-1 (IL-1), interleukin-6 (IL-6), and tumor necrosis factor-alpha (TNF-alpha), has been associated with accelerated bone loss and osteoporosis. These cytokines can increase the activity of osteoclasts, which are bone-degrading cells. There will be further bone resorption consequently [28].

ii. *RANKL and immune cells*: The receptor activator of the nuclear factor-kB ligand (RANKL) molecule is necessary for both osteoclast formation and bone resorption. Immune cells such as T cells and B cells can create RANKL, which promotes osteoclast activity. Immune system imbalances may cause an excessive amount of RANKL to be produced, which can lead to bone loss [28].

iii. *Autoimmune diseases*: Numerous autoimmune conditions that impair the immune system and are connected to an elevated risk of osteoporosis include systemic lupus erythematosus (SLE) and rheumatoid arthritis (RA). These conditions are brought on by the immune system attacking the body's own tissues specially the joints in the wrong way, which weakens the bones and leads to chronic inflammation [28].

iv. *Osteoporosis by glucocorticoids*: It is well-recognized that long-term use of glucocorticoids, such as prednisone, causes bone loss and increases the risk of developing osteoporosis. Glucocorticoids can affect the immune system, which can lead to aberrant bone remodeling, by reducing immune cell function and suppressing the production of pro-inflammatory cytokines [29].

v. *Lack of estrogen*: Osteoporosis is a major cause of estrogen loss after menopause since estrogen is necessary for maintaining bone health. Furthermore, estrogen has immunomodulatory effects, and immune system modifications brought on by estrogen deficiency may contribute to bone loss.

5. Potential immunological markers for osteoporosis diagnosis and prognosis

Numerous indicators may be able to predict the risk of fracture in osteoporosis. These include sphingosine-1-phosphate, sclerostin, periostin, macrophage migration inhibitory factor, and indicators of bone turnover. Additionally, it has been demonstrated that bone alkaline phosphatase and collagen-I-N-terminal propeptide can be used to predict the risk of fracture in older women.

5.1 Sphongosine-1-phosphate

Sphongosine-1-phosphate (S1P), a highly bioactive lysophospholipid that has been linked to a variety of biological processes including cell migration, localization, apoptosis, proliferation, and differentiation, has been shown to play a role in both extracellular and intracellular communication. S1P receptors (S1PRs) are expressed by osteoblasts as well as osteoclasts. Osteoblast survival, proliferation, and motility are stimulated by S1P, which osteoclasts release. The fascinating thing about S1P is that it is abundant in the bloodstream but is degraded irreversibly by S1P phosphatase and/or S1P lyase, leaving it low in other tissues. This assumes that S1P would be a viable biomarker predictive of phenotypes associated with osteoporosis because of this easily measured blood characteristic [30, 31].

5.2 Leucine-rich repeat-containing 17

A 37 kDa protein called leucine-rich repeat-containing 17 (LRRc17) has a secretary feature and five putative LRR domains. LRRc17, which is abundantly expressed in osteoblasts, inhibited NFATc1 signaling from RANKL-mediated activated T-cells, which therefore attenuated osteoclast genesis from BM precursors [32, 33].

5.3 Macrophage migration inhibitory factor

Macrophage migration inhibitory factor (MIF) is a 37.5 kDa cytokine that interacts with CD74 to have a variety of biological effects. Along with playing a role in the control of immunological and inflammatory processes. MIF has become a significant figure in bone metabolism [31, 33].

5.4 Sclerostin

Sclerostin is a protein that is secreted, largely by osteocytes, and whose concentration rises with aging. Sclerostin is a dual action molecule that negatively affects skeletal homeostasis by increasing bone resorption and decreasing bone formation. It also increases the development of osteocyte-derived RANKL. In order to support the notion that sclerostin is the perfect biomarker of human bone metabolism, various epidemiologic investigations have been conducted [31].

5.5 RANKL

RANKL plays essential roles at every stage of osteoclastogenesis and bone resorption. Although RANKL is expressed in various cell types, including osteoblasts, conditional genetic deletion indicates that osteocytes are the major source of RANKL needed for osteoclast formation [33].

5.6 Periostin

The extracellular matrix protein periostin, which contains glutamate, was first discovered in mouse pre-osteoblast MC3T3-E1 cells. It was given the name osteoblast-specific factor 2 at that time. Periostin is advantageous for bone metabolism, according to studies done on genetically modified mice [33].

6. Current treatment approaches for osteoporosis

The most popular treatments right now are anti-resorptive ones, which concentrate on stopping or slowing down the process of bone resorption. These medications include monoclonal antibodies, bisphosphonates, selective estrogen receptor modulators (SERMs), and estrogens.

Bisphosphonates are drugs that slow the loss and disintegration of bone (also known as resorption). They are frequently utilized in the management of osteoporosis. Alendronate, risedronate, ibandronate, and zoledronic acid are a few of the bisphosphonates that are commonly prescribed.

Hormone levels, particularly those of estrogens, play a significant role in bone resorption. SERMs have improved in their ability to lessen the adverse effects of estrogens. Although they can maintain bone mineral density (BMD) and show selectivity toward estrogen receptors in the bone, they are not as effective as conventional estrogens. Numerous clinical studies with postmenopausal osteoporotic women utilizing various SERMs have demonstrated that their value for fracture prevention is physically limited (present certain restrictions in preventing non-vertebral fractures). As well as having negative extra-skeletal effects, SERMs are also linked to related side effects such thromboembolic events and, in certain circumstances, carcinogenesis. These effects include a higher risk of cardiovascular events and endometrial cancer. The most popular anti-resorptive medications are bisphosphonates. Because of its affinity for hydroxyapatite, pyrophosphate analogues known as bisphosphonates attach to hard bone. They are absorbed by osteoclasts and integrated into the bone matrix, which inhibits their activity in bone remodeling. In this manner, bone density rises, but the quality of the bone is compromised since the aged bone is more likely to experience microfractures that impair its functionality. Additionally, long-term usage of bisphosphonates might result in unfavorable effects such as musculoskeletal discomfort, atrial fibrillation, osteonecrosis of the jaw, and gastrointestinal issues [34].

Denosumab is a monoclonal antibody that binds to the receptor activator of nuclear factor kappa-B ligand (RANKL) with a high affinity. By limiting the interaction of RANKL and RANK, the osteoclasts' ability to differentiate and function is inhibited. Regular adherence to Denosumab medication is a major worry because the patient's fracture risk could go up after the dose wears off. Another monoclonal antibody, Romosozumab, was just given the go-ahead by the US Food and Drug Administration to treat osteoporosis in postmenopausal women. It is the first humanized anti-sclerostin monoclonal antibody that has been demonstrated to increase bone formation with a dual effect. It does so by increasing bone formation while also, albeit to a lesser extent, reducing bone resorption (or bone loss), which lowers the risk of fracture [34, 35].

The existing osteoporosis treatments do not work completely in all individuals and have a number of adverse effects that substantially jeopardize their long-term efficacy. Thus, with a population that is aging and living longer, there is a need for the creation of novel therapeutic approaches for osteoporosis. However, there are some of the emerging therapies for osteoporosis.

Romozumab: A humanized monoclonal antibody called romozumab suppresses sclerostin. Sclerostin, a protein released by osteoclasts in the skeletal tissue, prevents osteoblasts from proliferating and functioning normally, hence reducing bone production [36]. Odanacatib: Odanacatib is a protease that selectively inhibits CatK, a protease that osteoclasts produce to hasten the breakdown of collagen in bones. It is hypothesized that inhibiting CatK will reduce bone resorption without reducing bone growth.

Lasofoxifene: A third generation SERM is lasofoxifene (Sermonix) [37, 38].

7. Conclusions and future directions

The primary goal of this book chapter is to deliver about the fragility fractures, which cause significant morbidity and impairment. In summary, osteoporosis is a complicated, chronic bone disease that has a big impact on health, finances, and society. Osteoporosis affects quality of life mostly through pain and functional limits, and it is predicted that in the coming years, its prevalence will increase dramatically. The delicate balancing act between bone formation and resorption that underlies the pathophysiology of osteoporosis is controlled by a number of immune cells, cytokines, and communication pathways. Osteoimmunology, a new subject, emphasizes the delicate relationship between bone health and the immune system. Both lymphoid and myeloid immune cells have a role in bone maintenance and remodeling. In the maintenance of bone homeostasis, specific functions are played by macrophages, dendritic cells, neutrophils, NK cells, ILCs, T cells, B cells, and regulatory B cells. The development of osteoporosis and bone loss can result from the dysregulation of these immune cells and inflammatory chemicals. To enhance the management of osteoporosis, new therapeutic modalities are being investigated. Monoclonal antibodies that target particular molecules, such as RANKL and sclerostin, have the potential to change the dynamics of bone remodeling. Protease inhibitors and third generation SERMs are further possible substitutes for traditional treatments. Future study into the immunological systems underlying osteoporosis is essential for creating cutting-edge therapeutic approaches. More individualized methods might result from the discovery of specific immunological markers for early diagnosis and prognosis. Immunotherapy, which focuses on controlling immune responses to improve bone health, has promise as a novel treatment option.

As our knowledge of the interaction between the immune system and bones grows, novel therapeutic approaches may be developed that will change the treatment of osteoporosis and enhance the lives of millions of people who are impacted by the disease.

Author details

Riya Mukherjee[1,2], Chung-Ming Chang[2,3*] and Ramendra Pati Pandey[4*]

1 Graduate Institute of Biomedical Sciences, Chang Gung University, Taiwan, Republic of China

2 Biotechnology Industry, Chang Gung University, Taiwan, Republic of China

3 Department of Medical Biotechnology and Laboratory Science, Chang Gung University, Taiwan, Republic of China

4 School of Health Sciences and Technology (SOHST), UPES, Uttarakhand, India

*Address all correspondence to: cmchang@mail.cgu.edu.tw
and ramendra.pandey@gmail.com

References

[1] Sietsema D. Fighting the epidemic: Bone health and osteoporosis. Nursing Clinics of North America. 2020;**55**(2):193-202. DOI: 10.1016/j.cnur.2020.02.002

[2] Rodrigo L. Introductory chapter: Osteoporosis overview. In: Osteoporosis—Recent Advances, New Perspectives and Applications. Spain: IntechOpen; 2021

[3] Hillier TA et al. WHO absolute fracture risk models (FRAX): Do clinical risk factors improve fracture prediction in older women without osteoporosis? Journal of Bone and Mineral Research. 2011;**26**(8):1774-1782. DOI: 10.1002/jbmr.372

[4] Rosen CJ. The Epidemiology and Pathogenesis of Osteoporosis—Endotext—NCBI Bookshelf. The Epidemiology and Pathogenesis of Osteoporosis—Endotext—NCBI Bookshelf. 2020. Available from: https://www.ncbi.nlm.nih.gov/books/NBK279134/

[5] Rodrigo L. Introductory Chapter: Osteoporosis Overview. Spain: IntechOpen; 2021. DOI: 10.5772/intechopen.97760

[6] Langdahl B, Ferrari S, Dempster DW. Bone modeling and remodeling: Potential as therapeutic targets for the treatment of osteoporosis. Therapeutic Advances in Musculoskeletal Disease. 2016;**8**(6):225-235. DOI: 10.1177/1759720X16670154. Epub 2016 Oct 5

[7] Ponzetti M, Rucci N. Updates on Osteoimmunology: What's new on the cross-talk between bone and immune system. Frontiers in Endocrinology. 2019;**10**:236. DOI: 10.3389/fendo.2019.00236

[8] Gong L, Zhao Y, Zhang Y, Ruan Z. The macrophage polarization regulates MSC osteoblast differentiation *In vitro*. Annals of Clinical and Laboratory Science. 2016;**46**(1):65-71

[9] Saxena Y, Routh S, Mukhopadhaya A. Immunoporosis: Role of innate immune cells in osteoporosis. Frontiers in Immunology. 2021;**12**:687037. DOI: 10.3389/fimmu.2021.687037

[10] Rivollier A, Mazzorana M, Tebib J, Piperno M, Aitsiselmi T, Rabourdin-Combe C, et al. Immature dendritic cell Transdifferentiation into osteoclasts: A novel pathway sustained by the rheumatoid arthritis microenvironment. Blood. 2004;**104**(13):4029-4037. DOI: 10.1182/blood-2004-01-0041

[11] Chakravarti A, Raquil MA, Tessier P, Poubelle PE. Surface RANKL of toll-like receptor 4-stimulated human neutrophils activates Osteoclastic bone resorption. Blood. 2009;**114**(8):1633-1644. DOI: 10.1182/blood-2008-09-178301

[12] Buckley MG, Walters C, Wong WM, Cawley MI, Ren S, Schwartz LB, et al. Mast cell activation in arthritis: Detection of alpha- and Beta-Tryptase, histamine and eosinophil cationic protein in synovial fluid. Clinical Science. 1997;**93**(4):363-370. DOI: 10.1042/cs0930363

[13] Soderstrom K, Stein E, Colmenero P, Purath U, Muller-Ladner U, de Matos CT, et al. Natural killer cells trigger Osteoclastogenesis and bone destruction in arthritis. Proceedings of the National Academy of Sciences of the United States of America. 2010;**107**(29):13028-13033. DOI: 10.1073/pnas.1000546107

[14] Luo G, Li F, Li X, Wang ZG, Zhang B. TNFalpha and RANKL promote

Osteoclastogenesis by upregulating RANK *via* the NFkappaB pathway. Molecular Medicine Reports. 2018;**17**(5):6605-6611. DOI: 10.3892/mmr.2018.8698

[15] Tang M, Tian L, Luo G, Yu X. Interferon-gamma-mediated Osteoimmunology. Frontiers in Immunology. 2018;**9**:1508. DOI: 10.3389/fimmu.2018.01508

[16] Wang T, He C. TNF-alpha and IL-6: The link between immune and bone system. Current Drug Targets. 2020;**21**(3):213-227. DOI: 10.2174/1389450120666190821161259

[17] Tanaka K, Hashizume M, Mihara M, Yoshida H, Suzuki M, Matsumoto Y. Anti-Interleukin-6 receptor antibody prevents systemic bone mass loss *via* reducing the number of osteoclast precursors in bone marrow in a collagen-induced arthritis model. Clinical and Experimental Immunology. 2014;**175**(2):172-180. DOI: 10.1111/cei.12201

[18] Srivastava RK, Sapra L. The rising era of "Immunoporosis": Role of immune system in the pathophysiology of osteoporosis. Journal of Inflammation Research. 2022;**15**:1667-1698. DOI: 10.2147/JIR.S351918

[19] Huang R, Wang X, Zhou Y, Xiao Y. RANKL-induced M1 macrophages are involved in bone formation. Bone Research. 2017;**5**:17019. DOI: 10.1038/boneres.2017.19

[20] Italiani P, Boraschi D. From monocytes to M1/M2 macrophages: Phenotypical vs. functional differentiation. Frontiers in Immunology. 2014;**5**:514. DOI: 10.3389/fimmu.2014.00514

[21] Swiecki M, Colonna M. The multifaceted biology of Plasmacytoid dendritic cells. Nature Reviews. Immunology. 2015;**15**(8):471-485. DOI: 10.1038/nri3865

[22] Nathan C. Neutrophils and immunity: Challenges and opportunities. Nature Reviews. Immunology. 2006;**6**(3):173-182. DOI: 10.1038/nri1785

[23] Artis D, Spits H. The biology of innate lymphoid cells. Nature. 2015;**517**(7534):293-301. DOI: 10.1038/nature14189

[24] Srivastava RK, Sapra L. The rising era of "Immunoporosis": Role of immune system in the pathophysiology of osteoporosis. Journal of Inflammation Research. 2022;**15**:1667-1698. DOI: 10.2147/JIR.S351918

[25] Wang S, Xia P, Chen Y, et al. Regulatory innate lymphoid cells control innate intestinal inflammation. Cell. 2017;**171**(1):201-216.e18. DOI: 10.1016/j.cell.2017.07.02

[26] Takayanagi H, Ogasawara K, Hida S, et al. T-cell-mediated regulation of osteoclastogenesis by signalling cross-talk between RANKL and IFN-γ. Nature. 2000;**408**(6812):600-605. DOI: 10.1038/35046102

[27] Ono-Ohmachi A, Yamada S, Uno S, et al. Effector memory CD4+T cells in mesenteric lymph nodes mediate bone loss in food-allergic enteropathy model mice, creating IL-4 dominance. Mucosal Immunology. 2021;**14**(6):1335-1346. DOI: 10.1038/s41385-021-00434-2

[28] Fischer V, Haffner-Luntzer M. Interaction between bone and immune cells: Implications for postmenopausal osteoporosis. Seminars in Cell & Developmental Biology. 2022;**123**:14-21. DOI: 10.1016/j.semcdb.2021.05.014. Epub 2021 May 20

[29] Briot K, Roux C. Glucocorticoid-induced osteoporosis. RMD Open. 2015;**1**(1):e000014. DOI: 10.1136/rmdopen-2014-000014

[30] Romero Barco CM, Arija SM, Pérez MR. Biochemical markers in osteoporosis: Usefulness in clinical practice | Reumatología Clínica. Biochemical Markers in Osteoporosis: Usefulness in Clinical Practice Reumatología Clínica; Spain. 2001. DOI: 10.1016/j.reumae.2011.05.004

[31] Rosen H, Goetzl EJ. Sphingosine 1-phosphate and its receptors: An autocrine and paracrine network. Nature Reviews. Immunology. 2005;**5**:560-570

[32] Kim BJ, Lee SH, Koh JM. Potential Biomarkers to Improve the Prediction of Osteoporotic Fractures. South Korea: PubMed Central (PMC); 2020. DOI: 10.3803/EnM.2020.35.1.55

[33] Kim D, LaQuaglia MP, Yang SY. A cDNA encoding a putative 37 kDa leucine-rich repeat (LRR) protein, p37NB, isolated from S-type neuroblastoma cell has a differential tissue distribution. Biochimica et Biophysica Acta. 1996;**1309**:183-188

[34] Srivastava RK, Dar HY, Mishra PK. Immunoporosis: Immunology of osteoporosis—Role of T cells. Frontiers. Apr 5 2018;**9**:657. DOI: 10.3389/fimmu.2018.00657

[35] Macías I, Alcorta-Sevillano N, Rodríguez CI, Infante A. Osteoporosis and the potential of cell-based therapeutic strategies. MDPI. 28 Feb 2020;**21**(5):1653. DOI: 10.3390/ijms21051653

[36] Zhang L, Yang Y, Geng D, Wu Y. Identification of potential therapeutic targets and molecular regulatory mechanisms for osteoporosis by bioinformatics methods. BioMed Research International. 10 Mar 2021;**2021**:1-0. DOI: 10.1155/2021/8851421

[37] Tafaro L, Napoli N. Current and Emerging Treatment of Osteoporosis. 2nd ed. Cham (CH): Springer; Chapter 15. 2021. DOI: 10.1007/978-3-030-48126-1_15. Available from: https://www.ncbi.nlm.nih.gov/books/NBK565567/

[38] Bolamperti S, Villa I, Rubinacci A. Bone remodeling: An operational process ensuring survival and bone mechanical competence—Bone research. Nature. 18 Jul 2022;**10**(1):48. DOI: 10.1038/s41413-022-00219-8

Chapter 4

Evaluation of *Plinia cauliflora* Effect in the Prevention of Osteoporosis in Ovariectomized Rats

Maxuel Fidelis de Padua Almeida, Guilherme Donadel, Mariana Dalmagro, Gabriel Maciel, Gabriela Zanuto de Lima, Marcia Alessandra Arantes Marques, Salviano Tramontin Bellettini, Ezilda Jacomassi, Giuliana Zardeto, Emerson Luiz Botelho Lourenço and Daniela de Cassia Faglioni Boleta Ceranto

Abstract

Osteoporosis (OSP) decreases bone mass and affects millions of people; the diagnosis is often late. Considering the side effects of conventional treatments, search for natural therapies should be a constant. Among natural treatments, herbal medicines stand out with very promising results. One of the plants that has drawn a lot of attention to prevent OSP is *Plinia cauliflora* (PC) Kausel. The objective was to evaluate the effect of PC extract in the OSP prevention in ovariectomized rats. In total, 60 female Wistar rats were divided into six experimental groups: positive control, negative control, sham, and three groups to test different doses (37.5, 75, and 150 mg) of PC bark extract. Bone mineral density (BMD), bone mineral content (BMC), hormone dosage, and osteocalcin were evaluated. One of the regions evaluated was the legs, where prolonged treatment with extract of PC in 75 mg, had a gain of 1.4 times of BMC. The levels of osteocalcin were found to be high at the lowest dose (37.5 mg), increasing the BMC by 70%, and moderately increasing the levels of dehydroepiandrosterone, proving that the pathway that increases BMC is through osteocalcin. PC resulted in increased BMC related mainly to increased osteocalcin, at the lowest dose preserving the bone matrix.

Keywords: osteoporosis, phytotherapeutics, animal model, bone mineral density, jabuticaba, osteocalcin

1. Introduction

Osteoporosis (OSP) is an ancient pathology, first observed in Egypt in 990 before Christ [1]. With the aging population in Brazil, the prevalence of osteoporosis has been increasing [2]. It causes more than 8.9 million fractures per year worldwide, without previous symptoms [3].

It is a systemic, progressive, and silent disease, with osteometabolic character [2]. Physiological processes occurs permanent bone remodeling throughout the patient's life. This process is altered in osteoporosis due to an increase in resorption and reduction of bone formation, causing it to lose its structural integrity, due to the cortical bone being porous and thinner [4].

This structural loss is responsible for the most common sign in osteoporotic individuals, which are bone fractures caused even by low impact [5] most frequently in the spine, distal radius, and proximal femur. Hip fractures are the most severe bringing a mortality of 12–20%, and about 50% of survivors of the condition of proximal femur fracture are unable to have an independent life [6].

OSP is effectively diagnosed by bone densitometry. However, the sensitivity of the method is low for assessing fracture risk, so there is no indication for population screening in menopausal women [7]. Due to the high prevalence of secondary causes of osteoporosis, one of the main examples being post-menopausal osteoporosis, characterized by hypoestrogenism can directly influence the proliferation and differentiation of osteoblasts, leading to changes in the levels of bone remodeling markers [8]. Several bone remodeling markers, especially those synthesized by osteoblasts (such as osteocalcin), are clinically used as predictors of postmenopausal osteoporosis. Unlike other biochemical markers of bone metabolism, osteocalcin can increase in all conditions in which there is bone remodeling, such as during childhood, after bone fractures or after osteoporosis induced by estrogen deficiency [9].

Osteocalcin, is a protein that plays an important role in bone mineralization, originates from osteoblastic synthesis and is deposited in the bone or released into the circulation, where it correlates with histological measures of bone formation [10]. In addition, osteocalcin can activate monocyte differentiation, resulting in an increase in the number of active bone resorption cells and promoting osteoclastic differentiation [11].

It is recommended for all patients, before starting any treatment, a laboratory evaluation that includes complete blood count, calcium, phosphorus, alkaline phosphatase, thyroid function, serum 25 (OH) vitamin D, 24-hour calciuria, and osteocalcin, as well as radiography of the thoracic and lumbar spine and proximal femur [12], dehydroepiandrosterone (DHEA), estradiol, and testosterone.

In view of the multifactorial nature of OSP, it is necessary that professionals are willing to treat, evaluate, and consider all the factors involved. For example, lifestyle changes, such as reduced smoking, healthy eating, and physical exercise [13], are essential for a better prognosis.

In some cases, not only a change in lifestyle will be enough to control and/or prevent the development of the disease but the introduction of specific drugs becomes indispensable.

Regarding the drug therapy used for the treatment and prevention of OSP, there are several classes, with major side effects, such as breast cancer, ovarian cancer, endometrial cancer, muscle damage, and a higher incidence of thrombosis. Due to the severe adverse effects, there is a need to seek natural alternatives for the treatment and prevention of OSP.

The jabuticaba (*Plinia cauliflora* (PC) Kausel) is native to South America, more precisely to the mountainous region around Rio de Janeiro and Minas Gerais in Brazil; as well as around Santa Cruz, Bolivia; Asunción, Paraguay and Northeastern Argentina. The fruits when ripe are highly nutritious and are mainly consumed as fresh fruits, but are also processed to make juice, wine, candy, liquor, ice cream, jams, and jellies [14].

One of the main actions of this plant is its function as a natural antioxidant, due to the anthocyanins of the flavonoid group, which have the characteristic to inhibit the oxidation of free radicals, protect, and stimulate collagen-rich tissues [15].

Quercetin presents an antioxidant effect and is within the group of flavonoids [16]. This antioxidative function inhibits the reaction of free radicals in osteoblastic cells, thus allowing the formation of bone matrix.

In addition to having antioxidant effects, they also have effects on hormone regulation through binding to steroids. The synthetic isoflavone that belongs to ipriflavone, within the metabolism of flavonoids, increases and aids in the maintenance of bone density in postmenopausal women [17].

In view of the above, the aim of the present work was to evaluate the effect of different doses of the bark extract of *P. cauliflora* in the treatment and prevention of osteoporosis in rats.

2. Material and methods

2.1 Animals

In total, 90-day-old female Wistar rats weighing between 250 and 300 g were randomized and housed in plastic cages with environmental enrichment at 22°C ± 2°C under a 12 h/12 h light-dark cycle and 55% ± 10% humidity. The animals had access *ad libitum* to food and water. All experimental procedures were reviewed by the Research Ethics Committee of Paranaense University (Protocol 37086/2020), and conducted according to the National Institutes of Health Guide for the Care and Use of Laboratory Animals (NIH Publications No. 8023).

2.2 Experimental design

Sixty rats distributed in 6 groups of 10 animals were used. The rats were anesthetized intramuscularly with ketamine (80 mg/kg) and xylazine (10 mg/kg). Forty animals underwent bilateral ovariectomy (OVX) (OVX groups). For OVX, the skin and muscles were incised longitudinally and the ovaries were identified and extirpated. The suture of the muscle layer was performed com single # 4.0 catgut threads, and the skin was sutured with # 4.0 nylon (Ethicon-Johnson & Johnson, São José dos Campos, SP, Brazil). Ten animals were subjected to sham OVX to simulate surgical stress (sham group). After exposing the ovary, it was removed from the abdominal cavity and after this procedure, the muscle layer and skin were sutured as described above. After surgery, all animals received enrofloxacin (10 mg/kg, subcutaneous, single dose) and ibuprofen (15 mg/kg, oral, once a day for 3 days) for infectious prophylaxis and analgesia, respectively. The rats also received 2 mL of saline solution subcutaneously for hydration. The surgical wound was cleaned with iodine and hydrogen peroxide once a day until complete healing.

Thirty days after surgery, the animals were divided into six groups (n = 10/group). There was a sham-operated group (fake operated to simulate surgical stress) (sham) and a negative control (NC) (which did not undergo any surgical procedure). The remaining ovariectomized animals were randomly included in the groups: positive control (OVX), and treatment with *Plinia cauliflora* in different doses: OVX + PC1 (37.5 mg/kg), OVX + PC2 (75 mg/kg) and OVX + PC3 (150 mg/kg). All animals underwent initial bone densitometry, 30 days after the surgery. For the densitometry examination, the animals were sedated with an intraperitoneal injection of 5 mg/kg diazepam.

The animals in the positive control (OVX), negative control (NC), and sham groups received vehicle (filtered water) daily in a volume of 5 mL/kg. The animals in the other groups (treatment) received the following doses of *Plinia cauliflora*: 37.5, 75, and 150 mg/kg, administered by oral wash (GO) once daily for 45 days. The animals were weighed weekly for regular dose adjustments.

The sequence of the experimental protocol is shown in **Figure 1**.

2.3 Drugs and solvents

Diazepam was obtained from Cristália (Itapira, SP, Brazil). All other reagents were obtained in analytical grade.

2.4 Obtaining the standardized extract of *Plinia cauliflora*

The aqueous extracts of *P. cauliflora* were obtained by infusion, using the fruit peel, as recommended by popular use [18] with minor modifications. The dried and ground plant extract (100 g) was submitted to the extraction process by infusion with 1 L of boiling water. The extraction was performed, for approximately 5 h, until the extraction medium reached room temperature. The solid residue (plant drug) was separated by filtration and the extract obtained was concentrated in a rotary evaporator to a volume of 200 mL.

The final product obtained was treated in a proportion of 1:3, that is, 600 mL of ethanol to 100 mL of the infusate so that the precipitation of proteins and polysaccharides occurs, secondary metabolites that arouse little interest in our area of studies. In this way, an ethanolic precipitate of the infuse (PEI) was obtained, which was

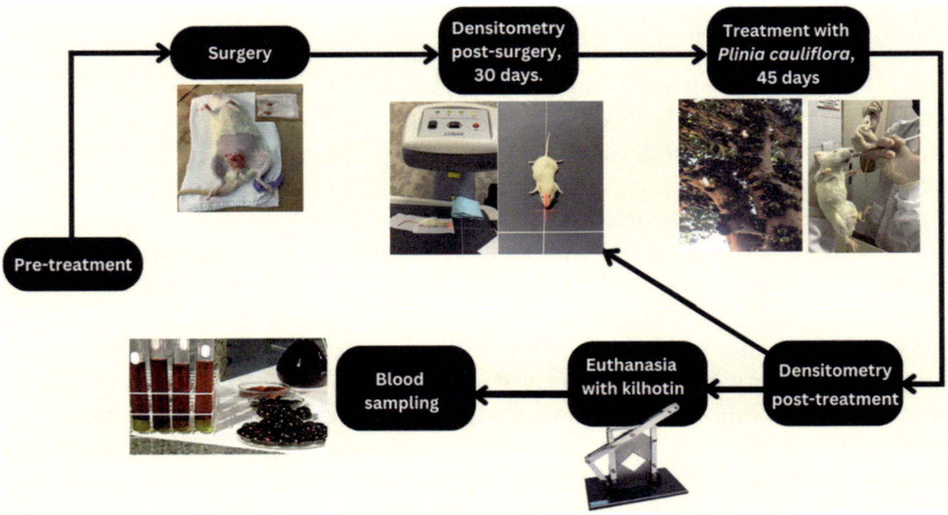

Figure 1.
Sequence of the experimental design.

discarded, and an ethanolic supernatant of the infuse of *P. cauliflora* (SEIPC). The SEIPC obtained was lyophilized and stored in a freezer (−20°C) until use.

2.5 Doses of the extract for the experimental set

The PC doses (37.5, 75, and 150 mg/kg) that were used in this study were calculated from the studies performed with atherosclerosis models by our research group with the same standardized extract [19].

2.6 Evaluation of serum levels of estradiol, progesterone, and DHEA

At the end of the experiments, the animals were euthanized by decapitation for total serum collection. Blood samples were collected in tubes containing ethylenediaminetetraacetic acid (EDTA) to obtain plasma. For analysis, serum was obtained by centrifugation (800 g, 10 minutes, 4) and stored at −20°C until analyzed. Estradiol and progesterone levels were determined by chemiluminescence immunoassay. DHEA levels were measured using an enzyme-linked immunosorbent assay. Serum osteocalcin levels were measured by electrochemiluminescence on an automated photomultiplier analyzer (PMT).

2.7 Bone mineral density measurements

Bone densitometry was performed using DXA (Lunar iDXA; General Electric, Boston, MA, USA) with software specially developed for small animals. Total body scanning was performed and total bone mineral density (g/cm^2) and bone mineral content (g) were analyzed. This scan was performed at two different times during the experiment: (1) 30 days post-OVX and (2) 45 days post-PC. The reason that bone mineral density was assessed after 30 days post-OVX was due to the significant bone loss that is typically observed [20]. For DXA, animals were sedated intraperitoneally with 5 mg/kg diazepam.

2.8 Statistical analysis

Results were expressed as the mean ± standard error of the mean of n = 6 animals per group. Statistical analyses were performed using one-way analysis of variance followed by Dunnett's test or Tukey's test. Values of $P < 0.05$ were considered statistically significant. Graphs were prepared and statistical analyses were performed using Prism 5.0 software (GraphPad, San Diego, CA, USA).

3. Results

3.1 Image parameters per DXA device

3.1.1 Validation of an imaging model of osteoporosis induced by ovariectomy

After 30 days of the ovariectomy procedure, the first measurement of total body composition was performed. When analyzed in general, considering all the body areas evaluated, a similarity was observed in the density and bone mineral content of all groups (**Figure 2**).

After the first densitometry, the groups were treated with the respective doses for a period of 45 days. Then a new measurement of the total body composition was

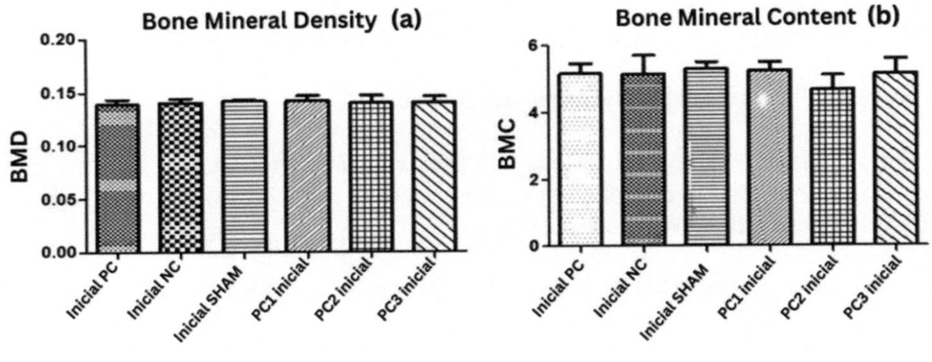

Figure 2.
*Total bone mineral density (g/cm²) (a) and bone mineral content (g) (b) after 30 days of performing ovariectomy (*p < 0.05; **p < 0.01; ***p < 0.001). Using one-way ANOVA followed by t-test. OVX: ovariectomized; NC: negative control; sham: sham ovariectomized; OVX + PC1: extract 37.5 mg/kg, OVX + PC2: extract 75 mg/kg; OVX + PC3: extract 150 mg/kg).*

made. When analyzed in general, considering all the body areas evaluated, a similarity was observed in the density and bone mineral content of all groups, however, the ovariectomized groups had a significantly lower increase than the sham group (**Figure 3a**). Regarding the bone mineral content, there was no significant difference in overall body bone mineral content between the groups evaluated (**Figure 3b**).

3.1.2 Evaluation of bone mass in pelvis and leg

Considering that densitometry evaluates parameters in different body regions and that the areas to evaluate osteoporosis through this exam in humans are lumbar spine and distal hip and radius, we chose to evaluate data in these regions alone. Although the prolonged treatment with standardized extract of *P. cauliflora* was not able to maintain the bone mineral content of the pelvis, it had an expressive positive result in the leg region, in the three doses evaluated (**Figure 4**).

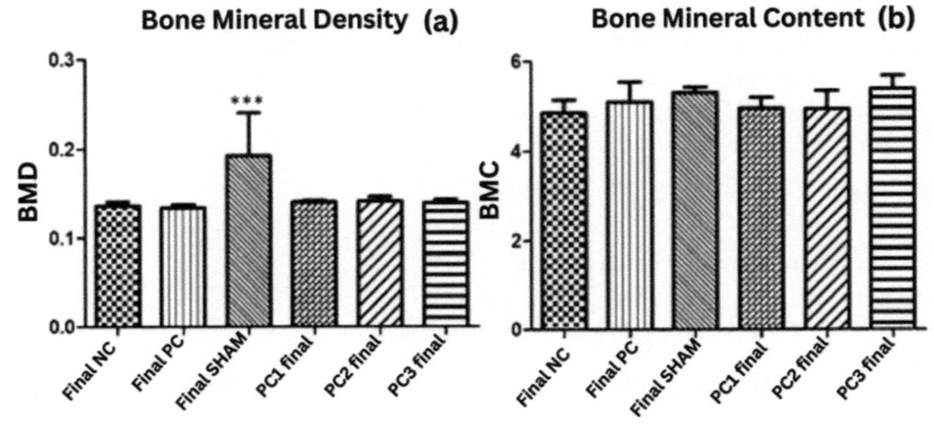

Figure 3.
*Total bone mineral density (g/cm²) (a) and bone mineral content (g) (b) after 45 days of instituted treatment (*p < 0.05; **p < 0.01; ***p < 0.001). Using one-way ANOVA followed by T-test. OVX: ovariectomized; NC: negative control; sham: sham ovariectomized; OVX + PC1: extract 37.5 mg/kg, OVX + PC2: extract 75 mg/kg; OVX + PC3: extract 150 mg/kg).*

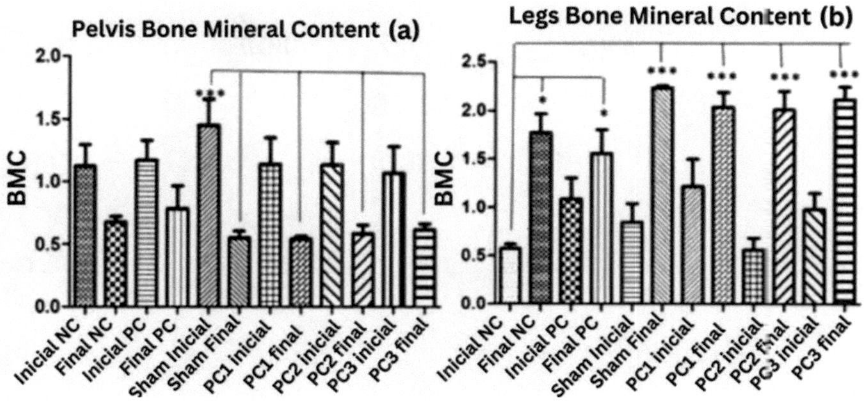

Figure 4.
*Bone mineral content (g) of pelvis (a) and leg (b) after 45 days of instituted treatment (*p < 0.05; **p < 0.01; ***p < 0.001). Using one-way ANOVA followed by t-test. OVX: ovariectomized; NC: negative control; sham: sham ovariectomized; OVX + PC1: extract 37.5 mg/kg, OVX + PC2: extract 75 mg/kg; OVX + PC3: extract 150 mg/kg).*

3.1.3 Evaluation of bone mass in the trunk

An interesting result was the dose-dependent effect found in the groups treated with sequential doses of *Plinia cauliflora* in the trunk region. As expressed in **Figure 5**.

3.1.4 Hormonal analyses

Serum estradiol and progesterone levels in the ovariectomized groups were significantly lower than in the sham group. Prolonged treatment with CP at all three doses significantly elevated serum osteocalcin levels and moderately elevated DHEA levels, without significantly altering estradiol or progesterone levels. The analyses also showed preservation and maintenance of bone turnover in the PC-treated groups compared with the sham operation group (**Figure 6**).

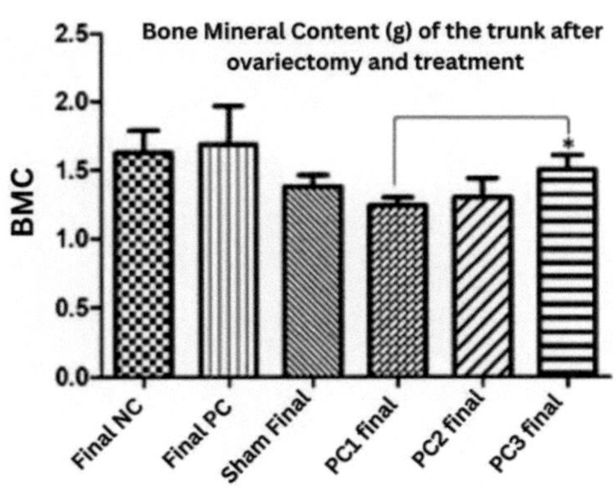

Figure 5.
*Bone mineral content (g) of the trunk after 45 days of instituted treatment (*p < 0.05; **p < 0.01; ***p < 0.001), demonstrating a dose-dependent effect in increasing bone content. Using ANOVA unidirectional followed by the t-test. OVX: ovariectomized; NC: negative control; sham: sham ovariectomized; OVX + PC1: extract 37.5 mg/kg, OVX + PC2: extract 75 mg/kg; OVX + PC3: extract 150 mg/kg).*

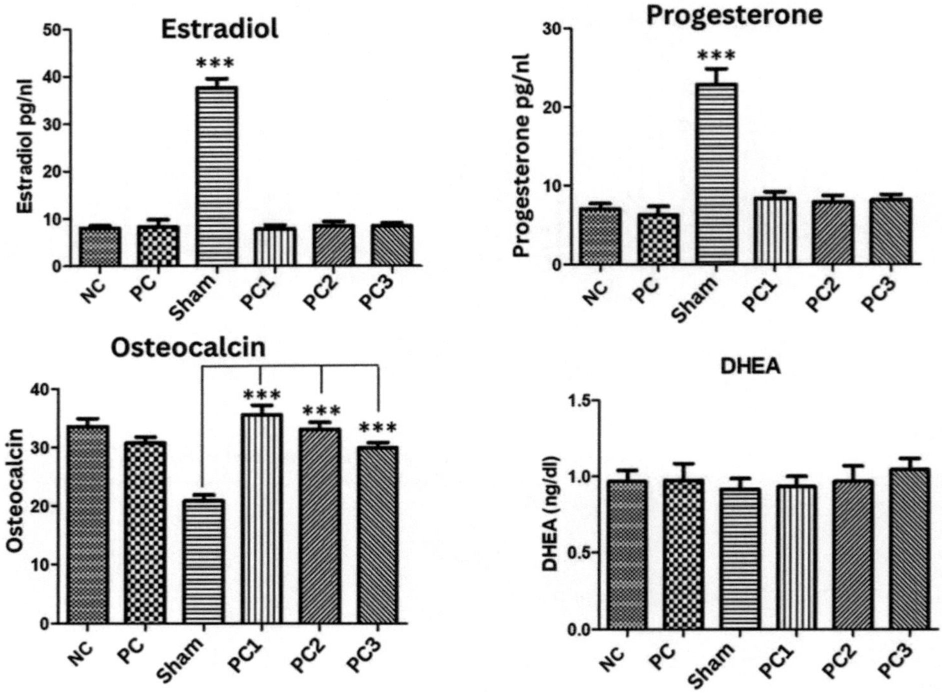

Figure 6.
*Serum levels of (a) estradiol (pg/ml), (b) progesterone (ng/dl), (c) DHEA (ng/ml), and (d) osteocalcin in the groups after 45 days of treatment (*p < 0.05; **p < 0.01; ***p < 0.001). Using one-way ANOVA followed by Tukey's test. OVX: ovariectomized; NC: negative control; sham: sham ovariectomized; OVX + PC1: extract 37.5 mg/kg, OVX + PC2: extract 75 mg/kg; OVX + PC3: extract 150 mg/kg).*

3.1.5 Histological analysis

The histological analysis of the tibiae showed the following results as shown in **Table 1**.

The OVX, sham, and OVX + PC1 groups developed 25%, 33.3%, and 40% osteoporosis, respectively. Animals in groups OVX + PC2 and OVX + PC3 did not develop osteoporosis in tibiae.

Groups	OSP (%)	Cell restoration (%)	Simple regeneration (%)	Tissue regeneration (%)
NC	0	100	0	0
OVX	25	75	0	0
sham	33.33	66.6	0	0
OVX + PC1	40	60	0	0
OVX + PC2	0	66.6	0	33.33
OVX + PC3	0	66.6	0	33.33

OVX: ovariectomized; NC: negative control; sham: sham ovariectomized; OVX + PC1: extract 37.5 mg/kg, OVX + PC2: extract 75 mg/kg; OVX + PC3: extract 150 mg/kg).

Table 1.
Percentage of bone changes in the different groups after oral administration of Plinia cauliflora (PC) extract standardized doses.

Cell restoration, which consists of reconstitution by own cells of disintegrated organelles, allowing them to survive and recover their functional capacity, occurred in 100% of the animals in the NC group, in 70% of the animals in the PCO group, 60% of the animals in the OVX + PC1 group, and in 66.6% in those in the sham, OVX + PC2, and OVX + PC3 groups.

Of the animals that received *P. cauliflora* at doses of 75 and 150 mg/kg, 33.33% developed tissue regeneration that is dependent on blood supply.

No group showed simple repair or scarring, which is the replacement of destroyed structures, without possibility of restoration, by elements of the regional support framework, in this case, a considerable increase in mineralization and fewer viable cells.

4. Discussion

Osteoporosis (OSP) is a systemic and silent disease, which generates an important oxidative stress in its pathophysiology. In recent years, there has been a significant increase in prevalence, due to the increased life expectancy of the population and also due to new medical technologies to make a more accurate diagnosis [1].

There are several classes of medications for OSP, with different mechanisms of action. Some of them act in increasing bone mass, others in preventing fractures, or, in the most current classes, allow the success of these two projections in the same medication. However, it is important to note that the side effects that these drugs can be significant, as some have the potential to cause irreversible adverse effects. This risk arises not only from the inherent properties of the drug, but also from the patient's clinical condition and the metabolic changes associated with aging [21]. It is worth emphasizing that osteoporosis is more prevalent among the elderly, and comorbidities tend to be more pronounced in this population.

One of the impacting factors in this pathology is the socioeconomic conditions of our country, since the classes of these medications have quite high values, often leaving patients without access to treatment. However, alternative medicine has been gaining shape to assist in the treatments, thus decreasing the adverse effects and even the costs of medication, making them more accessible to the population, without losing the effectiveness and the goal of the final treatment.

Among the herbal medicines, there are several alternatives that can help in the prevention and treatment of osteoporosis. One of the species that draws attention for its properties is the *Plinia cauliflora* (jabuticaba), a typical plant in our country.

Although the peels are generally discarded, according to the phytochemical study, they are rich in ellagic acid, quercetin (flavonoids), and anthocyanins, representing a great potential in antioxidant action [19].

Cells with higher levels of mitochondria are considered to have higher energy generation capabilities. RANKL-induced osteoclastogenesis results in increases in the size and number of mitochondria. In osteoporosis, this process is in a disorganized manner generating significant oxidative stress. Due to the antioxidant potential that *P. cauliflora* presents, it is hypothesized that it may control this bone resorption process [22].

Previous work by our group [2] demonstrated that in 30 days, there was a significant bone loss, which was not observed in the present study, considering the bone structure as a whole. Although no differences were observed in the general bone structures evaluated (BMD and BMC), as shown in **Figure 2**, when specific regions were compared, such as pelvis and legs, which represent the bone areas of greatest impact in rodents, significant differences were observed, mainly in the legs, in relation to bone mineral content, as observed in **Figure 4**, demonstrating the potential of *Plinia cauliflora* as a protective agent of this loss.

Because *Plinia cauliflora* is a plant extract from a fruit, which is considered a phytocomplex, and not an allopathic drug, it is more difficult to define exactly which active ingredients are responsible for the results obtained. However, the proposed model promoted a protective effect on bone loss in specific regions.

If we consider the cumulative effect of the plant's use over the period of the onset of diagnostic bone loss, we can suggest that in the long term, it has a positive impact on stemming the loss and consequently controlling the development of bone diseases such as osteoporosis.

The jabuticaba presents effects in the protection and stimulation of tissues rich in collagen and osteoblastic cells, helping in the formation of the bone matrix, in its two characteristics, both in the inorganic formation through the antioxidant actions on the ions, and in the organic formation, in which 95% is formed by collagen type 1, the union of these two formations generates a greater resistance to the bone. Within the inorganic formation, we find hydroxyapatite and calcium, two important ions for the formation of the bone matrix. Osteocalcin (OC) is responsible for fixing these two ions in the extracellular matrix thus affecting bone mineralization, therefore, OC is an important marker of osteoporosis [23].

Elevated levels of this protein (OC) during the absence of estrogen may indicate increased bone turnover. Since the main role of OC is bone mineralization, the body's calcium levels can profoundly alter its production and homeostasis. Calcium metabolism is very important during postmenopausal osteoporosis, the close relationship between reduced estrogen levels and bone loss may be directly related to this ion [11]. In the present study, it was observed that the three evaluated doses of *P. cauliflora* were able to increase the levels of OC, which can be hypothesized as a protective factor of bone mineral density, and in the highest dose (150 mg/kg), there was a 70% increase of bone mineral density.

Likewise, as the general structures of BMC and BMD were evidenced, the dosages of all hormones, including osteocalcin, which is a more expressive marker of bone mass loss, were analyzed quantitatively, that is, the total analysis of the animals was included, and not separately in the bone structures, where we verified the protective factor in the studied model. Additionally, a dose-dependent trend toward a protective response of PC against osteocalcin was observed, as illustrated in **Figure 6**.

P. cauliflora may be promising in the sense that it not only aids in cellular matrix formation but also in preventing bone loss. After the analysis of bone mineral content, we observed that treatment with the PC at three doses equaled the sham group and the control group, showing the effect of prevention against the loss of bone mineral content. The likely route of action of *Plinia cauliflora* for this result was through osteocalcin and not due to DHEA, which would be the most common route, due to the relationship that the sex hormone part presents in postovariectomy bone mineralization. Despite the effects already attributed to CP, its use had not yet been correlated to bone metabolism.

Other studies using extracts of *Tropaeolum majus* and *Tribulus terrestris* demonstrated protective bone effects when there is a decrease in urinary calcium with preservation of osteocalcin levels [11]. In Ref. [2], the authors evaluated the effect of *Tribullus terrestris* using the same methodology as the present study and demonstrated that increased bone mass was related to increased DHEA, respectively.

The works described in the literature correlate the increase of DHEA as an important factor in the increase of bone mass [24]. The decrease in DHEA is strictly related to changes found in postmenopause such as decrease in bone mass, decrease in muscle mass, increase in body fat accumulation, and diabetes mellitus [25]. However, the results of the present study demonstrated that *Plinia cauliflora*, at the three doses evaluated, despite having increased bone mass, the increase in DHEA levels was not significant, which leads us to suggest that the protective effect presented by *Plinia cauliflora*, and even bone mass gain, especially in the leg regions, may have been due to a greater impact generated in this region, a bone mass gain of 140% in the average dose (75 mg), through the osteocalcin pathway.

Study [26] revealed that OC is important in the process of alignment of collagen fibers parallel to hydroxyapatite, which would increase bone strength in long bones, and could justify the results of the present work. OC has a correlation with the formation of bone matrix, which is a precursor of mature osteoblastic cells, being one of the main markers of osteoblastic activity. Importantly, osteocalcin is an essential marker of bone matrix formation and not resorption, because it is completely destroyed by osteoclasts; its function is not well defined yet. However, studies indicate that its structure has an interaction with calcium and hydroxyapatite crystals and that its increase coincidentally correlates with the beginning of the mineralization process [27].

It has already been shown that 3-O-methyl gallic acid has the potential to prevent osteoporosis [28]. This molecule significantly suppressed osteoclast formation by blocking Akt and Btk-PLCγ2-Ca2+ signaling. Considering that *Plinia cauliflora* is rich in ellagic acid, a derivative of gallic acid, it is justified that the results obtained in bone protection may be related to the role of this compound in reducing osteoclasts.

Therefore, the antioxidant action that *Plinia cauliflora* presents through its chemical constituents, such as anthocyanins, ellagic acid, and quercetin, protect the osteocalcin pathway to act in the formation of bone mineralization, using in a more significant way the osteoblasts.

Although the effects attributed to *P. cauliflora* may be due to the increase in osteocalcin, after analysis of the trunk of the animals (rats), we observed that the three doses resulted in an equalization of bone mass gain, with the highest therapeutic dose PC3 (150 mg/kg/day) showing a more significant increase of 22% compared to the dose PC1. Therefore, it is possible that there are other osteoprotection mechanisms correlated to the extract since it is a phytocomplex from the peel of the *Plinia cauliflora* fruit, and thus there may be an increase in bone mass without correlation with the increase in hormones, for example, changes in inflammatory cytokines and antioxidant enzymes.

5. Conclusion

Treatment with *Plinia cauliflora* extract resulted in improved bone mineral density. The results suggest that this increase is not related to DHEA or sex hormones but to the increase of osteocalcin. The elevation of osteocalcin preserved the bone matrix after 45 days of treatment in ovariectomized rats. The three doses evaluated maintained an equal pattern for the prevention of matrix loss, suggested to be the probable responsible for the osteoporosis prevention effects. In the model used, it should be considered that the protection analysis was evaluated over a period of 45 days against the proposed treatment groups, but it should be taken into account that osteoporosis, being a chronic disease, can manifest itself more intensely over longer periods, which is suggested to be analyzed in future studies, in different periods. Further work is needed to evaluate its role as a protective agent in this experimental model. Additional preclinical and clinical studies may clarify the mechanism of action of this natural product in the treatment and prevention of osteometabolic diseases.

Conflict of interest

"The authors declare no conflict of interest."

Author details

Maxuel Fidelis de Padua Almeida, Guilherme Donadel, Mariana Dalmagro, Gabriel Maciel, Gabriela Zanuto de Lima, Marcia Alessandra Arantes Marques, Salviano Tramontin Bellettini, Ezilda Jacomassi, Giuliana Zardeto, Emerson Luiz Botelho Lourenço and Daniela de Cassia Faglioni Boleta Ceranto*
Paranaense University, Umuarama, Brazil

*Address all correspondence to: dcboleta@prof.unipar.br

References

[1] Bucholz RW et al. Fraturas em Adultos de Rockwood & Green. 7th ed. Barueri, SP: Manole; 2013. 492-590 pp

[2] Marques MAA, Lourenço BHLB, Reis MDP, Pauli KB, Soares AL, Belettini ST, et al. Osteoprotective effects of Tribulus terrestris L.: Relationship between dehydroepiandrosterone levels and Ca2+-sparing effect. Journal of Medicinal Food. 2019;**22**(3):241-247. DOI: 10.1089/jmf.2018.0090

[3] Pisani P, Renna MD, Conversano F, Casciaro E, Di Paola M, Quarta E, et al. Major osteoporotic fragility fractures: Risk factor updates and societal impact. World Journal of Orthopedics. 2016;**7**(3):171-181. DOI: 10.5312/wjo.v7.i3.171

[4] Amadei SU, Silveira VÁS, Pereira AC, Carvalho YR, Rocha RFD. A influência da deficiência estrogênica no processo de remodelação e reparação óssea. Jornal Brasileiro de Patologia e Medicina Laboratorial. 2006;**42**:5-12. DOI: 10.1590/S1676-24442006000100003

[5] Lee DR, Lee J, Rota M, Lee J, Ahn HS, Park SM, et al. Coffee consumption and risk of fractures: A systematic review and dose-response meta-analysis. Bone. 2014;**63**:20-28. DOI: 10.1016/j.bone.2014.02.007

[6] Orwig DL, Chan J, Magaziner J. Hip fracture and its consequences: Differences between men and women. Orthopedic. Clinics. 2006;**37**(4):611-622. DOI: 10.1016/j.ocl.2006.08.003

[7] Wannmacher L. Manejo racional da osteoporose: onde está o real benefício. Organização Pan-Americana da Saúde/ Organização Mundial da Saúde-Brasil; 2004. pp. 1-7. DOI: 10.1055/S-0033-1346697. Available from: https://core.ac.uk/download/pdf/48116592.pdf

[8] Swaminathan R. Biochemical markers of bone turnover. Clinica Chimica Acta. 2001;**313**(1-2):95-105. DOI: 10.1016/S0009-8981(01)00656-8

[9] Bikle DD. Biochemical markers in the assessment of bone disease. The American Journal of Medicine. 1997;**103**(5):427-436. DOI: 10.1016/S0002-9343(97)00137-X

[10] Atalay S, Elci A, Kayadibi H, Onder CB, Aka N. Diagnostic utility of osteocalcin, undercarboxylated osteocalcin, and alkaline phosphatase for osteoporosis in premenopausal and postmenopausal women. Annals of Laboratory Medicine. 2012;**32**(1):23-30. DOI: 10.3343/alm.2012.32.1.23

[11] Barboza LN, Prando TBL, Dalsenter PR, Gasparotto FM, Gasparotto F, Jacomassi E, et al. Prolonged diuretic activity and calcium-sparing effect of *Tropaeolum majus*: Evidence in the prevention of osteoporosis. Evidence-Based Complementary and Alternative Medicine. 2014. Article ID 958291. DOI: 10.1155/2014/958291

[12] Papaioannou A, Morin S, Cheung AM, Atkinson S, Brown JP, Feldman S, et al. Clinical Practice Guidelines for the Diagnosis and Management of Osteoporosis in Canada: Background and Technical Report. Canada, Ontario: Scientific Advisory Council of Osteoporosis; 2010. Available from: https://osteoporosecanada.ca/wp-content/uploads/Osteoporosis_Guidelines_2010_Background_And_Technical_Report.pdf

[13] Marques MAA, Lima DA, Andreotti CE, Junior AG, ELB L. Caracterização das plantas medicinais e medicamentos fitoterápicos para tratamento da osteoporose utilizados

no Brasil. Arquivos de Ciências da Saúde da UNIPAR. 2016;**20**(3):183-188. DOI: 10.25110/arqsaude.v20i3.2016.5870

[14] Lin CY, Yin MC. Renal protective effects of extracts from guava fruit (*Psidium guajava* L.) in diabetic mice. Plant Foods for Human Nutrition. 2012;**67**:303-308. DOI: 10.1007/s11130-012-0294-0

[15] Maia JL. Desenvolvimento de microcápsulas contendo as antocianinas presentes no corante do extrato do jambo por polimerização interfacial [thesis]. Natal, RN: Universidade Federal do Rio Grande do Norte; 2013. Available from: https://repositorio.ufrn.br/handle/123456789/15845

[16] Knekt P, Isotupa S, Rissanen H, Heliövaara M, Järvinen R, Häkkinen S, et al. Quercetin intake and the incidence of cerebrovascular disease. European Journal of Clinical Nutrition. 2000;**54**(5):415-417. DOI: 10.1038/sj.ejcn.1600974

[17] Knight DC, Eden JA. Phytoestrogens-a short review. Maturitas. 1995;**22**(3):167-175. DOI: 10.1016/0378-5122(95)00937-G

[18] Lorenzi H, Matos FJA. Plantas Medicinais no Brasil: Nativas e Exóticas. 2ª ed. Instituto Plantarum: Nova Odessa; 2008

[19] Romão PVM, Palozi RAC, Guarnier LP, Silva AO, Lorencone BR, Nocchi SR, et al. Cardioprotective effects of Plinia cauliflora (Mart.) Kausel in a rabbit model of doxorubicin-induced heart failure. Journal of Ethnopharmacology. 2019;**242**:112042. DOI: 10.1016/j.jep.2019.112042

[20] Lelovas PP, Xanthos TT, Thoma SE, Lyritis GP, Dontas IA. The laboratory rat as an animal model for osteoporosis research. Comparative Medicine. 2008;**58**(5):424-430. Available from: https://www.ncbi.nlm.nih.gov/pmc/articles/PMC2707131/

[21] Wimalawansa SJ, Razzaque MS, Al-Daghri NM. Calcium and vitamin D in human health: Hype or real? The Journal of Steroid Biochemistry and Molecular Biology. 2018;**180**:4-14. DOI: 10.1016/j.jsbmb.2017.12.009

[22] Park-Min KH. Metabolic reprogramming in osteoclasts. Seminars in Immunopathology. 2019;**41**(5):565-572. DOI: 10.1007/s00281-019-00757-0

[23] Zanatta LC, Boguszewski CL, Borba VZ, Kulak CA. Osteocalcina, metabolismo energético e da glicose. Arquivos Brasileiros de Endocrinologia & Metabologia. 2014;**58**:444-451. DOI: 10.1590/0004-2730000003333

[24] Jankowski CM, Gozansky WS, Schwartz RS, Dahl DJ, Kittelson JM, Scott SM, et al. Effects of dehydroepiandrosterone replacement therapy on bone mineral density in older adults: A randomized, controlled trial. The Journal of Clinical Endocrinology & Metabolism. 2006;**91**(8):2986-2993. DOI: 10.1210/jc.2005-2484

[25] Labrie F, Bélanger A, Bélanger P, Bérubé R, Martel C, Cusan L, et al. Metabolism of DHEA in postmenopausal women following percutaneous administration. The Journal of Steroid Biochemistry and Molecular Biology. 2007;**103**(2):178-188. DOI: 10.1016/j.jsbmb.2006.09.034

[26] Komori T. Functions of osteocalcin in bone, pancreas, testis, and muscle. International Journal of Molecular Sciences. 2020;**21**(20):7513. DOI: 10.3390/ijms21207513

[27] Vieira JGH. Considerações sobre os marcadores bioquímicos do metabolismo ósseo e sua utilidade prática. Arquivos Brasileiros de Endocrinologia & Metabologia. 1999;**43**:415-422. DOI: 10.1590/S0004-27301999000600005

[28] Baek JM, Kim JY, Lee CH, Yoon KH, Lee MS. Methyl gallate inhibits osteoclast formation and function by suppressing Akt and Btk-PLCγ2-Ca2+ signaling and prevents lipopolysaccharide-induced bone loss. International Journal of Molecular Sciences. 2017;**18**(3):581. DOI: 10.3390/ijms18030581

Chapter 5

Immunomodulation of Bone Remodeling in Osteoporosis

Sayantee Hazra, Shagnik Chattopadhyay and Ritobrata Goswami

Abstract

Reducing bone density and bone quality with increasing propensity of skeletal fracture are the main symptoms of osteoporosis. Disruption of the fine balance between bone formation and resorption leads to this progressive condition, which affects 50% of women and 30% of men after the age of 50. Aging, reduced nutrient (vitamin D and calcium) uptake, suppressed production of estrogen, and primarily, the dysregulation of cytokine balance leads to the pathophysiology of the disease. Hence, immunomodulation of bone remodeling is tightly controlled by the cytokine profiles, epigenetic marks, and metabolic programs of the involved cells, thus playing a key role in the prognosis of osteoporosis. In this chapter, we highlight this intricate interplay between the immune system, the associated cytokines, and bone remodeling.

Keywords: immunomodulation, epigenetics, cytokines, bone remodeling, immune cells

1. Introduction

In healthy people, bone is an active tissue that is constantly replenished, in great part thanks to the immune system. Numerous inflammatory bone disorders are connected to any imbalance between the processes of bone production and bone resorption. The immune system is crucial for both tissue growth and bone resorption. In addition to immune cells and cytokines, bone cells, such as osteoblasts (OBs), osteoclasts (OCs), and osteocytes (OSs), also have an impact on how immune cells function on a cellular level. As a result, the immune microenvironment plays a critical role in regulating the rate at which bones heal, mend, and regenerate.

OBs, OCs, OSs, and other fundamental components make up bone. As a dynamic organ, the skeletal system and immune system interact intricately, maintaining a balance between bone creation and bone resorption. In addition to coexisting in the bone marrow (BM) cavity, bone and immune cells also share a range of regulatory molecules and progenitor cells. The regulation of bone homeostasis by immune cells is known to be influenced by bone cells. Likewise, the proliferation and differentiation of immune cells is also modulated by bone cells. As a result, the term "osteoimmunology" was created to emphasize the interaction between the immunological and skeletal systems [1].

IntechOpen

The skeleton is a very dynamic structure that changes throughout the course of a person's life in order to maintain bone density and mineral homeostasis by continuously regenerating the bone matrix. The dynamic equilibrium that results from a succession of well-planned biological events—all of which are controlled by intricate interactions between the many cell types that are found in bone—is physiological bone remodeling. OBs and OCs are the primary cells involved in bone remodeling. Additionally, OSs, which operate as mechanical sensors, are crucial to the process of bone remodeling, whereas bone lining cells (BLCs) start the process by degrading the matrix. The five successive steps of the bone remodeling cycle are activation, resorption, reversal, formation, and termination [2].

An immune response is immediately triggered by tissue damage, and it typically lasts for days or even weeks. The two main effects of immune cells on bone regeneration are the catabolic effect of chronic inflammation during bone resorption and the anabolic effect of acute inflammation during bone regeneration. By encouraging the proliferation and osteoblastic differentiation of mesenchymal progenitor cells, acute inflammation, for instance, can result in the synthesis of chemokines that speed up bone formation during the early stages of bone fracture healing [3]. While an adaptive immune response is significant during late bone remodeling, an acute inflammatory response is essential at the start of bone regeneration. When the inflammatory response is under control, it can aid in bone regeneration; however, when the inflammation is out of control, it can be harmful to bone tissue. For an anabolic milieu that promotes bone growth and repair, the management of inflammation is essential.

This chapter delineates the immunological events leading to bone remodeling and the pathophysiology of osteoporosis. Detailed emphasis has been provided pertaining to the activity of immune cells leading to bone remodeling. Additionally, the chapter incorporates a separate section on the implication of bone generative and bone degenerative cytokines in bone remodeling. In the biological signal regulatory network, epigenetics primarily serves as a posttranscriptional controlling mechanism. The final section of the chapter discusses research developments on epigenetic mechanisms in the osteogenic differentiation and the pathogenesis of osteoporosis to provide a new direction for the treatment of diseases related to bone metabolism, considering the significant role of epigenetic mechanisms in the regulation of bone metabolism.

2. Bone remodeling and osteoporosis

2.1 Bone remodeling

Our bones encompass a vast and intricate network of connective tissue, which provides mechanical support (skeletal system), protects our internal organs, and forms a dais for smoother functioning of numerous bodily functions. Although primarily formed of inorganic calcium and phosphate, it is a site of living cells, tissue, and a complex network of highly active metabolic processes [4]. Despite being hard and resilient, bones can be exceptionally adaptive and can restructure themselves under varying mechanical forces and differential loading [5].

Bone remodeling can be defined as the spatiotemporally regulated physiological phenomenon, which involves de- and re-construction of bone matrix to ensure precise turnover and proper distribution of osteogenic tissue throughout the body of the organism. Bone resorption and formation are tightly conjoined to ensure that under

Sl no.	Components (by dry weight)		
	Organic (~30%)	Inorganic (~60–65%)	
1	Type 1 collagen	Hydroxyapatite crystals	Order of abundance
2	Osteopontin	Carbonate	
3	Bone sialoprotein	Potassium	
4	Bone acidic glycoprotein	Strontium	
5	Thrombospondin	Chloride	
6	Fibronectin	Fluoride	
7	Other non-collagenous proteins	Other trace minerals	
9	Water (10%)		

Table 1.
The different components of osteogenic tissue in order of their abundance [7].

homeostatic conditions, there is minimal loss of bone mass in a healthy individual [5]. Bone remodeling assists in cleaning up the circulating blood by absorbing the toxic chemicals (like drugs), radioactive debris, heavy metals, etc. by temporarily storing them in newly ossified matrix and slowly releasing it during the latter phases of deconstruction [6]. Ossified tissue also serves as a reservoir of two very important materials, namely calcium and phosphorus, and bone remodeling helps in maintaining a homeostatic level between the blood and the bone [6].

Bones, unlike other forms of connective tissue, consist of cells that make up the living organic matter, and the calcified matrix serves as the inorganic counterpart. The exact composition of the bone tissue is summarized in **Table 1**. Compact bones are involved in the bulk of skeletal structure supplying most attachment points for muscles and tendons, while cancellous bones are found along the inner layers of the compact bones and consist of trabeculae. These cancellous bones house the marrow, which is primarily involved in the metabolic and hematopoietic functions. Effective remodeling of the bone tissue requires the involvement of different types of cells, which together make up the most rudimentary functional structure called the BMU or basal multicellular unit [4] (**Figure 1**). BMUs primarily consist of BLCs, OBs, OSs, and OCs. At any given moment, there are about 1–2 million active BMUs engaged in remodeling, although they may be working asynchronously at different sites. Initial phases of bone remodeling ensure that BMUs can start excavating micro-tunnels along the poles of either the trabecular or cortical bones. This is followed by the bone resorption phase, which involves recruitment of giant multinucleate osteoclasts and decay of inner lining of the bone to form empty channels or tunnels called Howship's lacunae [4]. In the latter part of remodeling process, the function of OCs is restricted in a manner resembling the reversal of their initial activity. Osteoprogenitors and post-osteoclastic cells are recruited to the site of remodeling [4], and they start reforming the lining ("cementing line") of the lacunae, where new bone formation can take place. Additionally, the reabsorbed surfaces are cleaned up by the BLCs and resident macrophages. Finally, the differentiation of new osteoblasts from preosteoblastic mesenchymal stem cells takes place [8]. These osteoblasts restart ossification of the inner lining, as well as the mineralization of osteoid tissue that they have synthesized themselves. More importantly, tissue-resident immune cells, including B-cells, effector and regulatory T-cells, dendritic cells, natural killer cells, myeloid

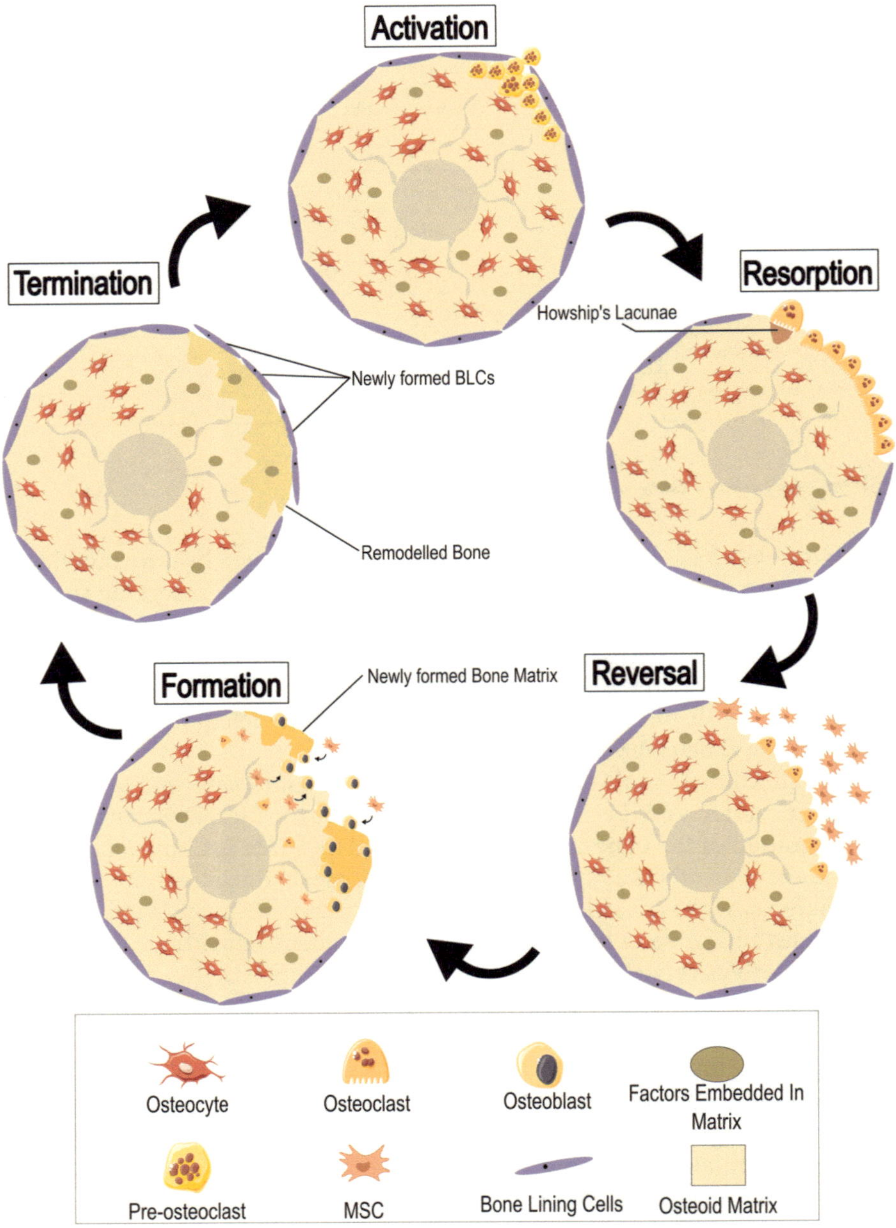

Figure 1.
Process of bone remodeling and bone turnover mediated in five distinct stages, namely; activation, resorption, reversal, formation, and termination. Each of these stages presents with unique features that have been highlighted. The first phase involves disruption of the BLC layer and infiltration of pre-osteoclastic stem cells, which differentiate into OCs. These OCs then start degrading the bone. The reversal phase witnesses the restricted activity of the OCs with the simultaneous influx of MSCs, differentiating into OBs. The OBs dominate the formation phase and finally transition into termination phase, whereby the BLCs reform and the cycle of bone remodeling ends.

cells, etc. also impact the bone remodeling to maintain the homeostatic environment [9]. Thus, BMUs complete one cycle of bone remodeling, ensuring that refilling of the excavated channels occurs smoothly [4].

2.2 Role of bone remodeling in osteoporosis

The word osteoporosis can be viewed as an assembly of two parts namely, "osteo" denoting bone and "poros" meaning pores or holes. Literally, the word translates to "holes in the bones". Hence, osteoporosis can be described as an assemblage of clinical conditions that primarily culminates into a significant decrease in bone density, skeletal deformity, and increased susceptibility to fractures. It is the most common form of bone disease in adults and over the age of 50 [10]. It is known to affect all genders and races, although females have higher disposition to develop this disease after menopause due to hormonal imbalance. This condition has no outright manifestations, and once detected, severely hampers the quality of life of the patients. In severe cases, it can result in other secondary complications and can even be the cause of mortality in patients. Affected individuals experience pain, inability to move freely, fractures from otherwise harmless impacts, and various physical restrictions.

Extensive bone remodeling occurs throughout the lifetime of an individual organism. As stated earlier, loss of osteogenic tissue is supplemented by the growth of new tissue, which ensures that there is no alteration in net bone mass [3]. A multitude of factors, including environmental, genetic, nutritional, hormonal, and physical strains, influence this bone formation and its shape. With aging, the degree of remodeling is affected and bone loss starts to occur. Various elements heighten this process of resorption over formation. This triggers fluctuations in the microarchitectural level, resulting in bone loss over time. Loss of individual trabecular bone plates structurally weakens the skeletal framework with significantly diminished bone density [8]. Evidently, this elevates the risk of fractures, which is further exacerbated by other age-related declines in bodily functions.

3. Factors affecting bone remodeling

The coordinated process of bone formation and degradation is regulated by various local and systemic factors in a well-synchronized manner. Apart from age, lifestyle, diet, and genetic background, there are plethora of factors that regulate this harmonious cycle. While parathyroid hormone, estrogen, progesterone, and androgen are the hormones, vitamin D (Vit D) and calcium form the major micronutrients to regulate the concert of the bone remodeling process through paracrine, autocrine, or endocrine actions. Several growth factors and cytokines also play a pivotal role in the bone remodeling cycle (**Figure 2**).

Apart from these factors, the immune system significantly impacts the regeneration and repair of osteogenic tissue. The ability of bone tissue to regenerate is determined by the immune microenvironment's role in bone tissue healing, repair, and regeneration. Disruption of this well-synchronized process aids in the development of several degenerative diseases, such as osteoporosis and osteoarthritis. Thus, immunologic modulations can be attributed to the maturation of osteoporosis, and the varied functions of the different immune cells, in this regard, can be correctly and collectively termed as "immunoporosis" [11, 12]. The detailed discussion on the role of hormonal factors, micronutrients, and growth factors are beyond the scope of this chapter. Here, our focus is on the immunoregulation of bone remodeling process and how it affects immunoporosis [12]. A comprehensive overview has been given in **Table 2**.

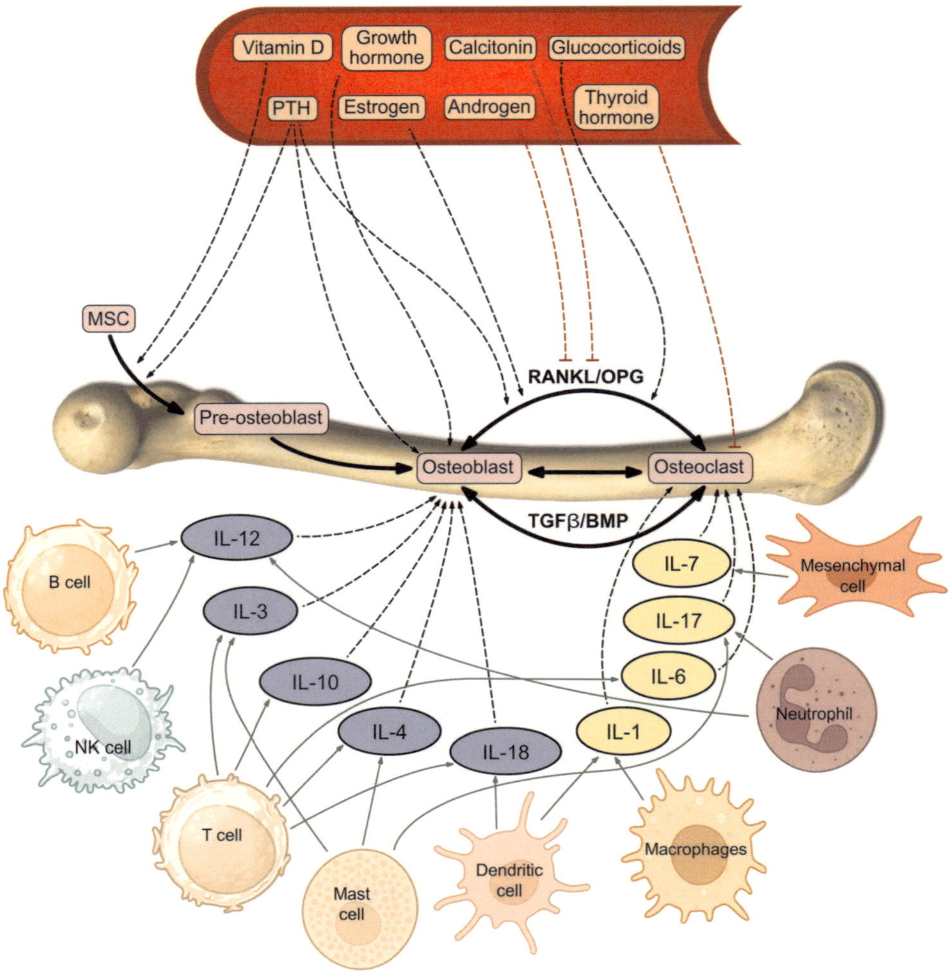

Figure 2.
The complex process of bone remodeling is governed by various cytokines, micronutrients, and hormonal factors. Immune cells, such as dendritic cells, macrophages, neutrophils, mesenchymal cells, and T cells, secrete cytokines, including IL-1, IL-6, IL-17, IL-7, etc., which play a crucial role in initiating the process of bone degeneration. Contrastingly, some cytokines such asIL-12, IL-3, IL-10, IL-4, IL-18 etc. contribute to osteoblastic differentiation.

4. Cytokines in bone remodeling

The mechanism of bone remodeling is a fine balance between bone regeneration and degeneration, which has been regulated by diverse factors. The cells present in the bone microenvironment, such as bone marrow stromal cells, OBs, OCs, macrophages, and T lymphocytes produce these peptide factors, which engages with several cell signaling pathway to directly or indirectly modulate the osteoclastogenesis and osteoblastogenesis processes. Even though most of the cytokines have biphasic impacts, we can still group them into two different classes: (a) bone regenerative cytokines and (b) bone degenerative cytokines. In the subsequent sections, we discuss them in more detail.

Type of regulators	Cytokines	Source	Receptors	Activated pathways	Target cells	Reference
Positive regulators	IL-3	Lymphoid cells, mast cells, eosinophils	IL-3R	JAK2/STAT5, NF-KB	Osteoblasts	[13]
	IL-4	Mast cells, Th2 cells, eosinophils, basophils	IL-4R	JAK/STAT6	Osteoblasts	[14]
	IL-10	Treg, Th2, monocytes, macrophages, dendritic cells, Bregs	IL-10R	RANK/OPG, NFATC1	Osteoblasts	[15]
	IL-12	Macrophages, neutrophils and B cells	IL-12R	RANK/OPG, NFATC1, FAS/FASL	Osteoblasts	[16]
	IL-13	Th2, mast cells, eosinophils	IL-13R	JAK/STAT6	Osteoblasts	[17]
	IL-18	Macrophages, dendritic cells, perhaps lymphocytes, and by nonimmune cells	IL-18R	FAS/FASL, nitric oxide pathway	Osteoblasts	[18]
	IL-19	Monocytes, dendritic cells	IL-20R	NF-κB, p38MAPK, c-FOS	Osteoblasts	[19]
	IL-27	Dendritic cells, macrophages	IL-27R	JAK/STAT1/STAT3, MAPK and NF-κB	Osteoblasts	[20]
	IL-29	Dendritic and macrophages	IL-28R1/IL-10R2	JAK/STAT	Osteoblasts	[21]
	IL-32γ	NK cells, T cells, monocytes	PR3	JAK/STAT3	Osteoblasts	[22]
	IL-33	Epithelial cells, fibroblasts, and endothelial cells, mast cells and dendritic cells	ST2	Bax, FAS/FASL	Osteoblasts	[23]
	IL-35	Dendritic, Treg cells, Bregs	IL-12R	JAK1/STAT1, NF-κB and MAPK	Osteoblasts	[24]
	IL-37	Monocytes, dendritic cells	IL-18R/IL-1R	PI3K/AKT	Osteoblasts	[25]
	IL-11	Osteoblasts, Bone marrow stromal cells	IL-11R	RANKL/OPG, Wnt	Osteoclasts	[26]
Negative regulators	IL-1	Tissue macrophages, monocytes, fibroblasts, and dendritic cells, B cells	IL-1/IL-1R1	NF-κB, MAPK	Osteoclasts	[27]
	IL-6	Monocytes, endothelial cells, and adipose tissue	IL-6R	P3IK/AKT, MAPK, and JAK/STAT	Osteoclasts	[28]
	IL-7	Mesenchymal and epithelial cells	IL-7R	c-Fos/c-Jun, AKT, STAT5	Osteoclasts	[29]

Type of regulators	Cytokines	Source	Receptors	Activated pathways	Target cells	Reference
	IL-8	Monocytes/macrophages, endothelial cells	IL-8R	RANKL/ OPG	Osteoclasts	[30]
	IL-15	Monocytes, macrophages, dendritic cells	IL-15R	ERK	Osteoclasts	[31]
	IL-17	Th17, neutrophils, microglia, mast cells	IL-17R	JNK, ROS and MEK/ ERK	Osteoclasts	[32]
	IL-20	T cells, B cells, NK cells, macrophages	IL-20R	JAK/STAT, NF-κB	Osteoclasts	[33]
	IL-34/ M-CSF	Endothelial cells, fibroblasts, osteoblasts, smooth muscle, and macrophages	IL-34R, CSF-1R	JAK/STAT3, NFATc1	Osteoclasts	[34]
	IL-23	Activated macrophages and dendritic cells	IL-23R	JAK/STAT	Osteoblasts/ osteoclasts	[35]

Table 2.
The growth factors and cytokines responsible for regulation of bone remodeling.

4.1 Bone regenerative cytokines

4.1.1 IL-3

Activated T lymphocytes, mast cells, and OBs producing this cytokine share its βc subunit of receptor with GM-CSF and IL-5 receptors. IL-3 inhibits osteoclastogenesis through different pathways. This cytokine blocks the RANKL-dependent NF-κB nuclear translocation process. It inhibits the phosphorylation of IκB of the RANKL-induced pathway in pre-OC cells, which prevents the further development of the OCs [36]. IL-3 also downregulates the expression of TNFRs (TNFR1 and TNFR2) on OCs to suppress TNF-dependent OC differentiation and bone degeneration process [37, 38]. The mRNA and protein levels of PU.1, c-FOS, and c-Fms also get downregulated substantially by IL-3, which, in turn, suppresses the maturation of bone monocytes and OC precursor cells [39–41]. It directly targets the OB-specific genes, such as alkaline phosphatase, collagen type-I, OCN, OPN, and some transcription factors, such as Runx-2 and OSX. This cytokine also targets JAK/STAT signaling pathway to promote OBs differentiation [42]. IL-3 has the capability to enhance RANKL expression, independent of OPG expression [13]. This cytokine governs two functional variants of RANKL by decreasing the activity of metalloproteinases, encompassing ADAM10, ADAM17, ADAM19, and MMP3, to lessen the expression of soluble RANKL and enhance the expression of membrane-bound RANKL. This modulation is carried out through the JAK2/STAT5 signaling pathway, thus reinstating the reduced RANKL-OPG ratio in adult mice [13].

4.1.2 IL-4

Th2 cells predominantly secrete this pleiotropic cytokine that acts as an immunomodulatory cytokine but also as a potent inhibitor of osteoclastogenesis. IL-4 also targets the phosphorylation of IκB to inhibit NF-κB translocation in a STAT6-dependent manner, which directly inhibits both OCs maturity and bone resorption activity [14]. Like IL-3, it also blocks RANKL and TNF-α-induced osteoclastogenesis *via* the MAPK signaling pathway [43]. IL-4 also suppresses transcription factors nuclear factor activated T cells c1 (NFATC1) of RANKL-induced signaling pathway through STAT6, which further inhibits OCs formation [44]. The endothelial cells present in the bone's vascular system release osteogenic cytokines and hormones that regulate the process of bone development, remodeling, and repair [45]. IL-4 and its closely associated counterpart, IL-13, can indirectly impede the formation of OCs by activating the STAT6 pathway. This activation prompts endothelial cells to release the hormone OPG, which is known for its role in safeguarding bone health [17] IL-4 is also indirectly involved in inducing osteoblastogenesis. RANKL, in the presence of M-CSF, induces OCs formation, but in the presence of GM-CSF and IL-4, the very same cocktail helps to induce the TNF-α converting enzyme, which further sheds the M-CSF receptor and stimulates the monocyte to differentiate into dendritic cells rather than OC cells [46].

4.1.3 IL-10

Th2 and Treg cells are the main sources of this anti-inflammatory cytokine. It acts as a direct inhibitor of the RANKL-OPG-RANK axis [15]. This cytokine induces OPG expression, which, in turn, blocks soluble RANKL from binding with RANK and further inhibits OCs differentiation [47]. IL-10 also suppresses RANKL-induced OCs maturation and calcium signaling through triggering receptors expressed on myeloid cells 2 [TREM-2] transcriptional inhibition [48]. IL-10 also suppresses NFATC1 expression through inhibition of c-Fos, and c-Jun nuclear translocation [49]. Apart from the details mentioned earlier, the reduced expression of IL-10 cytokines in individuals with osteoporosis serves as additional confirmation of its anti-osteoclastogenic characteristics [50]. Even studies with IL-10-deficient mice show lower bone mass, reduced bone formation, and increased bone fracture [51]. Regarding osteogenic differentiation, IL-10 restrains bone marrow osteogenic function by impeding bone mineralization in mouse bone marrow cells. Moreover, it hampers the production of bone proteins such as ALP, type I collagen, and OCN [52].

4.1.4 IL-11

Another important player in bone remodeling, this cytokine is also known as adipogenesis inhibitory factor [AGIF] [53]. It can modulate the osteoclastogenesis process in both RANKL-dependent and independent pathways [54]. Research has shown that mice with IL-11 overexpression exhibit thickened bone cortex, increased bone mass, and enhanced bone strength; while the IL-11R knockout mice are characterized by impaired bone formation and increased adipose in bone marrow. This study indicates the positive role of IL-11 in osteoblastogenesis [55]. Compared to this, additional studies have also claimed that IL-11 can also promote osteogenesis and inhibit adipogenesis through the WNT signaling pathway [3].

4.1.5 IL-19

This cytokine belongs to the IL-10 family as well, and it operates in a comparable fashion to its counterpart, IL-10. It keeps the OCs in their precursor state by targeting and suppressing NF-κB and p38MAPK activation and c-Fos expression [19]. IL-19 also blocks OC-specific RANKL pathways. Furthermore, it can enhance the release of osteoclastogenic cytokines such as IL-1β, IL-6, and TNF-α in osteoporosis conditions. However, little study has been done on how IL-19 affects osteoporosis [56].

4.1.6 IL-12

Functioning as an anti-osteoclastogenic cytokine, it hinders NFATC1 to impede osteoclastogenesis driven by RANKL [57]. IL-12 also stimulates FASL-dependent apoptosis in OB cells [16]. Along with IL-18, IL-12 also induces an OC apoptosis mechanism, which reveals the anabolic role of this cytokine in the bone remodeling procedure.

4.1.7 IL-18

IL-18 is a pro-inflammatory cytokine that operates in synergy with TNF-α and IL-12 and is responsible for stimulating the generation of nitric oxide. This, in turn, expedites the apoptosis process in osteoclast cells [18]. Furthermore, it stimulates T cells to produce IFN-γ and GM-CSF for inhibiting OC maturation indirectly [58]. Studies conducted using mice that have undergone ovariectomy (OVX), display that administering IL-18 binding protein (IL-18BP), which acts against IL-18, results in the restoration of bone loss [59]. Moreover, the observation of reduced IL-18BP levels in the serum of women with osteoporosis further suggests the role of IL-18 as a cytokine that promotes bone regeneration [56].

4.1.8 IL-13

Th2-specific anti-osteoclastogenic cytokine IL-13 acts in a very similar way to IL-4. It triggers the production of OPG through STAT6 activation to inhibit OCs proliferation [17]. Both IL-13 and IL-4 are capable of blocking OB cyclooxygenase-2 (COX-2)-dependent prostaglandin synthesis, which, in turn, inhibits bone resorption [60].

4.1.9 IL-27

IL-27 is a member of the IL-6/12 cytokine family. This bone-regenerating cytokine blocks RANKL-dependent c-Jun and NFATc1 expression *via* MAPK and NF-κB pathway. It also suppresses NFATc action by downregulating TREM2 expression [61]. Additionally, it inhibits OCs maturation in c-Fos-dependent manner [20]. IL-27 suppresses RORγt-dependent IL-17 differentiation and induces IL-10-producing Treg cell formation by activating Egr2 while inhibiting OBs apoptosis in a similar way [62]. Additionally, the findings on female osteoporosis patients suggest that the blood levels of the RANKL repressor Id2 got increased and that Egr2 and IL-27 levels dropped in comparison, demonstrating the anabolic role of IL-17 in the bone regeneration process [62].

4.1.10 IL-29

IL-29 is a family member of the interferon family, which activates the JAK/STAT signaling pathway. Dendritic cell producing this cytokine inhibits OC formation and bone degeneration both *in vivo* and *in vitro* [21]. Similar to other bone-regenerating cytokines, it also has RANKL-dependent OC maturation and blocks NF-κB activation, and NFATC1 translocation [63].

4.1.11 IL-33

IL-33, belonging to the IL-1 family, possesses osteoprotective capabilities unlike IL-1. It suppresses osteoclastogenesis by at least three mechanisms. IL-33 inhibits RANKL-dependent NFATC1 expression *via* the ST2 receptor pathway, which, in turn, suppresses osteoclast formation [64]. In a very similar way, it induces OCs apoptosis by increasing BAX, Fas, and FASL expression [23]. An *in vivo* study has confirmed that IL-33 stimulates the mRNA expression of bone regenerative cytokines such as IL-4, IL-10, IL-13, and GM-CSF [65]. It also synergistically acts with Vit D in the repression of the OCs maturation [66]. Research has also suggested that mice exhibiting elevated levels of TNF-α can experience recovery through IL-33 treatment [67]. Moreover, IL-33 encourages OBs activity, facilitates the deposition of matrix minerals, and decreases the levels of sclerostin mRNA in primary OBs subjected to prolonged ascorbate treatment [68]. According to a recent study, postmenopausal women with osteoporosis have significantly lower IL-33 levels than the healthy controls [69].

4.1.12 IL-35

This anti-inflammatory and immunosuppressive cytokine belongs to the IL-12 family, which directly inhibits OCs formation, TNF-induced osteoclastogenesis and bone resorption. IL-35 suppresses NFATC1, c-Fos, and TRAP *via* the NF-κB and MAPK pathways. By activating JAK1/STAT1, this action not only prevents the development of OCs produced by TNF but also promotes apoptosis [24]. IL-35 also shows an inhibitory effect on RANKL and M-CSF-induced Th17/IL-17 axis-regulated OC formation and bone degeneration [70]. Osteoporosis occurs due to the imbalance of bone and adipogenesis. MSCs have the ability to differentiate either in OBs or adipocyte cells. Research has found that IL-33 stimulates MSC differentiation toward OBs formation by inducing the expression of OB-specific factors, such as β-catenin and Axin2. It also suppresses the apoptosis of MSCs and differentiation into adipocyte cells [71]. In contrast, IL-33 was also found to induce phosphorylation of osteoclast-specific signaling molecules such as Syk, phospholipase Cγ2, Gab2, MAP kinases, TAK-1, and NF-κB and transcription factors such as TRAF6, NFATc1, c-Fos, C-Src, histone-K, and calcitonin receptor, which leads to bone resorption [72].

4.2 Bone degenerative cytokines:

4.2.1 TNF

TNF family, consisting of TNF-α and TNF-β, plays a significant bidirectional role in bone erosion. TNF stimulates OCs development, even *via* RANKL/RANK-independent axis. TNF-α initiates the activation of stromal cells and OBs. This cascade indirectly leads to the upregulation of RANK in OC precursors and subsequently promotes the process of OC formation through M-CSF [73]. Instead of activating the RANK/RANKL axis, TNF-α can induce OCs differentiation through the sequential activation of NF-κβ, p50/52, c-Fos, and NFATC1 [74, 75]. TNF-α can also trigger IL-1β production by pre-OC cells, which, in turn, stimulate differentiation of OC cells [76].

Tumor necrosis factor receptor-associated factors (TRAFs) play a significant role in bone remodeling. They possess the ability to initiate OCs formation in response to TNF. Notably, among these factors, TRAF6 holds the capacity to influence and regulate the process of osteoclastogenesis [77]. Some studies have demonstrated that RANKL might trigger the degradation process of TRAF3 to enhance the OCs differentiation process in TRAF-independent manner [78]. A lower concentration of TNF stimulates osteoblastogenesis, while a higher concentration strictly inhibits it. TNF also inhibits both bone regenerating factors IGF-1 and RUNX2 [79].

4.2.2 IL-1

The bone, degenerative cytokine IL-1 comprises of IL-1α and IL-1β. This class of cytokines induces osteoclastogenesis by activating OCs differentiation, multinucleation, and survival [80]. IL-1β has both direct and indirect effect on the bone remodeling process. It can indirectly boost the TNF-mediated osteoclastogenesis process in addition to directly upregulating RANKL synthesis to improve OC differentiation [81]. Through a process involving the elevation of M-CSF and PGE2 expression, as well as the concurrent downregulation of OPG expression in OBs, IL-1 has the capacity to induce the production of OCs-like cells (OLCs) [82]. IL-1 could trigger OCs differentiation in bone marrow-derived macrophages (BMMs) through a pathway that does not rely on the RANKL/RANK interaction. This occurs *via* IL-1/IL-1R1 signaling and involves the activation of genes associated with osteogeneses such as NF-κB, JNK, p38, ERK, and the microphthalmia transcription factor (MITF), which, in turn, induces the differentiation of OCs [27]. However, this mechanism does not increase the expression of c-Fos or NFATc1, which both must remain at a specific baseline level for this process to occur [27]. IL-1 not only induces OCs formation but also suppresses OCs maturation and has an impact on the bone fracture healing process [27].

4.2.3 IL-6

Secreted by OBs, bone marrow stromal cells, OCs, macrophages, and T cells, this pleiotropic cytokine transmits its signal through IL-6R, which is shared by a distinctive set of factors such as IL-11, oncostatin M (OSM), leukemia inhibitory factor (LIF), cardiotrophin (CT-1), ciliary neurotrophic factor (CNT)] cardiotropin such as cytokine factor 1 (CLCF1), neuropoietin (NP), IL-27, and humanin [28]. IL-6 can indirectly promote osteoclastogenesis by activating RANKL, which is produced by stromal and osteoblast cells, through JAK-mediated activation of STAT3 [83]. Study in murine model demonstrates that excessive IL-6 expression can result in increased OC development and decreased bone mass [84]. Another study using a mouse model lacking in IL-6 demonstrates an increase in tartrate-resistant acid phosphatase (TRAP), positive OCs cells, and elevated ALP activity in OBs [85]. Another experiment with IL-6-deficient mice also shows increased apoptosis in OC cells [86]. This study has revealed the osteoclastogenic regulatory role of IL-6. However, research has also reported the suppressive role of IL-6 on OCs formation through the suppression of the RANK signaling pathway-driven degradation of IκB and the initiation of JNK activation [87]. The role of IL-6 in bone remodeling depends not only on its own concentration but also on the presence of different concentrations of RANKL. IL-6/IL-6R mediates its suppression regulation process through NF-κB, ERK, and JNK [88]. Additionally, IL-6 knock-out mice experiments have demonstrated that genes controlled by OBs, such as Runx2 and Col1A1, are upregulated following ovariectomy, while OCs-related genes, such as TRAP, MMP9, and CTSK, are found to be downregulated [89]. The osteoporosis mouse model has shown that the IL-6/STAT3 pathway suppresses β-catenin activity and leads to increased inflammation reaction in the bone microenvironment, while the recovery from the disease progression has been achieved by using an anti-IL-6 antibody [90]. Furthermore, IL-6 prompts an elevation in the expression of TLR2, TLR4, IL-1, and TNF-α within BMSCs. This, in turn, triggers activation of the AKT pathway and subsequently leads to the suppression of Setd7 expression [91]. IL-6 also targets the activation of JAK/STAT, SHP2/MEK2, SHP2/AKT signaling pathway in OBs and induce their differentiation [92]. Interestingly, IL-6 has also been found to activate STAT3, signaling which promotes osteoclastogenic differentiation in an autocrine/paracrine feedback loop [91].

4.2.4 IL-7

In response to the IL-1 and TNF-α, OBs and stromal cells produce another IL-2 superfamily cytokine, IL-7. This cytokine indirectly promotes osteoclastogenesis by triggering T lymphocytes to produce RANKL and TNF-α [29]. Studies with IL-7 transgenic mice have shown lower bone mass and reduced osteoclastogenesis [93]. Additionally, it has been observed that the quantity of T lymphocytes affects the function of IL-7 in the bone microenvironment [29]. Research has substantiated that the lack of estrogen, post-OVX leads to increased IL-7 levels. This, in turn, encourages the thymus-dependent differentiation of bone marrow-derived progenitor cells and the thymus-independent peripheral expansion of mature T cells. Consequently, this process enhances the development of T lymphocytes and triggers bone loss [94]. Apart from T lymphocyte development, IL-7 is also involved in B lymphocyte development, which also plays a major role in bone resorption [95]. Recent studies propose that IL-7/IL-7R might oversee the distinct mechanisms involving CTSK, NFATc1, and MMP9, along with the phosphorylation events of p38 and Akt [96]. This is accomplished through the activation of the c-Fos/c-Jun pathway, thereby leading to an augmentation in the count of OCs and the extent of bone resorption in macrophages that are stimulated by RANKL [97]. Another study has suggested that IL-7 also has an anti-osteoclastogenic role in the presence of CSF-1 and RANKL [96]. However, additional details are not yet available.

4.2.5 IL-15

IL-15 is another member of the IL-2 superfamily. This cytokine also performs its role in a very similar way to IL-17. IL-15 exerts an indirect stimulating influence on the creation of OCs, acting in synergy with RANKL to primarily trigger OCs formation. This is primarily accomplished by activating the extracellular signal-regulated kinase (ERK) pathway, which enables this collaborative influence [31]. Another study of bone marrow and OBs co-culture has shown that IL-5 treatment may trigger OBs apoptosis [98].

4.2.6 IL-34

Like M-CSF, this cytokine also binds to the CSF-1R and triggers OCs regeneration and differentiation in the very same way as IL-34. In the presence of RANKL, this cytokine amplifies the process of osteoclastogenesis [99]. Few studies have elucidated the role of this cytokine in bone remodeling. One such research investigation revealed that IL-34 facilitates the growth and specialization of bone marrow macrophages into osteoclasts. This is achieved through an elevation in NFATc1 expression, the stimulation of p-STAT3 expression, and the suppression of Smad7 expression, all in the absence of M-CSF [34]. Furthermore, another research study reported that a low dosage of IL-34 enhances fracture healing *via* the PI3K/AKT and Erk pathways, yet it does not affect osteoclast formation *in vitro* [32].

4.2.7 IL-17

The secretion of this pro-inflammatory cytokine by Th17 cells has a pivotal function in bone immunology. A study involving mice with ovariectomy (OVX) demonstrated elevated IL-17 expression alongside an increased count of Th17 cells. This elevation fosters the production of osteoclastogenic cytokines, including TNF-α, IL-6, and RANKL, within osteoblast cells. Consequently, this process contributes to bone loss [32]. Estrogen or IL-17 treatment leads to a significant amount of bone loss, where anti-IL-17 antibody administration enhances the activity of FOXO1 and ATF4 to increase osteoblastogenesis [100]. In humans, the level of IL-17 increases after menopause and shows a significantly lower amount of minerals in bone [101]. In addition to stimulating the expression of RANKL, TNF-α, IL-1, IL-6, and IL-8 cytokines in osteoclasts (OCs), IL-17 also triggers autophagy in OC precursors. This, in turn, leads to the formation of OCs *via* JNK signaling, showing an association with lower concentrations [102]. However, research also shows the dose-dependent effect of IL-17 in bone remodeling. Increased concentration of IL-17 suppresses OCs differentiation and downregulates the MMP-9 and histone-K expression to inhibit matrix protein hydrolysis during bone resorption [103]. IL-17 triggers the upregulation of M-CSF and RANKL expression in hMSCs, facilitating the progression of OCs formation in both *in vitro* and *in vivo* [104]. Research has shown that IL-17 shows a positive effect on early OBs differentiation but an inhibitory effect on osteoblastic calcification [105]. *In vitro*, elevated levels of IL-17 prompt OBs impairment through the NLRP3 inflammatory vesicle pathway. This instigates the liberation of IL-1 and RANKL, further disturbing the equilibrium of bone metabolism [106].

4.2.8 IL-20

IL-20 is another IL-10 family cytokine, highly expressed in osteoporosis patient serum compared to normal patients. Treatment with anti-IL-20 antibody leads to the suppression of M-CSF and RANKL-induced OCs formation *in vitro* [33]. IL-20 triggers osteoclastic signals such as NF-κB, TRAF6, STAT3, NFATC1, and c-Fos. This cytokine has the capability to induce the expression of RANKL in both OBs and OCs [33]. Study has shown that IL-20 could hinder the viability and maturation of OBs by increasing the expression of sclerostin while decreasing the levels of OSX, RUNX2, and OPG [107].

4.2.9 IL-22

Th22 cell producing this cytokine is another member of IL-10 family and helps to defense and wound healing of intestinal epithelium and skin tissue. Research has indicated the elevated levels of IL-22 in the blood serum. The observation has also revealed that instead of IL-17 alone, IL-22 plays an immense role in osteoclast differentiation through MAPK phosphorylation [108].

4.2.10 IL-23

This cytokine induces osteoclastic proliferation by differentiating naïve Th cells into Th17 cells, which produce osteoclastogenic IL-17, to further bone degeneration [109]. This cytokine can also induce OCs formation by upregulating RANKL expression in the bone marrow and CD4+ T cells [35]. Nonetheless, the impact of IL-23 on bone within a living organism is also subject to debate. This uncertainty arises from a particular study's findings, which suggest that IL-23 indirectly impedes osteoclast development *in vitro* through a CD4+ T lymphocyte-dependent mechanism that is further contingent on the dosage employed [110].

5. Immune cells in bone remodeling

The immune system, which functions as a protective barrier against invasive diseases and bodily harm, is made up of a variety of cell types. The immune system is divided into two main sections: the innate immune system, which provides rapid protection, and the adaptive immune system, which is highly specific to antigens. Upon tissue damage, the initial responders are predominantly innate immune cells like neutrophils, macrophages, and dendritic cells. As the tissue damage continues, specific adaptive immune cells such as T and B cells, which are tailored to the antigens involved, are drawn to the site. Acute inflammation governs the bone regeneration phase, while chronic inflammation regulates the bone resorption phase within the process of bone remodeling. Given below are the immune cells that are pivotal in bone biology.

5.1 Neutrophils

Neutrophil is the prevailing form of polymorphonuclear phagocyte cell, typically being the initial innate immune cell to arrive at the site of injury [111]. These cells combat pathogens through phagocytosis and by generating reactive oxygen species (ROS) *via* the synthesis of granzyme B and perforins [112].

Numerous clinical and animal experiments have implicated the involvement of neutrophils at the bone erosion site. The increased level of inflammatory cytokines and elevated number of macrophages at the bone lesions site indicates the effect of neutrophils during the bone healing mechanism [113]. A recent study underscores the fact that neutrophils produce an emergency extracellular matrix-rich fibronectin to trigger the fracture healing process [114]. In contrast, some studies have reported the involvement of neutrophils in osteoclastogenesis. Recent research has reported that TLR4-activated neutrophils can produce a higher amount of cell membrane RANKL (m-RANKL), which is different from CD3+ lymphocyte-producing soluble RANKL [115]. The activated neutrophils' mRANKL affects both OCs and their mononuclear precursors, transforming them into fully developed and operational OCs that play a role in bone resorption [116]. Moreover, it has been noted that neutrophils augment the differentiation of OCs induced by vitamin D3 in co-culture setups involving bone marrow cells and OBs [117]. Additionally, neutrophils stimulate the breakdown of

OPG, leading to increased osteoclastogenesis in bone marrow cells [118]. To summarize, neutrophils balance bone homeostasis during early phase of bone injury.

5.2 Macrophages

Macrophages are recognized as the initial precursors of OCs. Circulating macrophages started to reside within the organs to become tissue-resident macrophages (TRM), such as osteocytes in bone. Distinct macrophage populations exist within the bone structure, including bone marrow macrophages (BMMs), OCs, and osteal macrophages, often referred to as "osteomacs." Osteomacs are observed near the OBs, offering anabolic assistance to these cells in terms of bone mineralization and the process of bone formation by releasing bone regenerating cytokines such as BMP-2, BMP-4, TGF-B1 [119]. Osteal macrophages play a major role in bone mineralization [120].

When exposed to a defined array of stimuli, immature macrophages can be categorized into two main classes: M1 macrophages, which are generally pro-inflammatory, and M2 macrophages, known for their anti-inflammatory properties [121]. Studies have shown that during early phase of bone injury, M1 macrophages can transdifferentiate into OCs followed by stimulated pro-inflammation [122]. An investigation using both the RAW 264.7 murine macrophage cell line and bone marrow-derived macrophages (BMDMs) highlights the fact that M1 macrophages induced by lipopolysaccharide (LPS) and IFN-γ, notably hinder RANKL-induced osteoclastogenesis by releasing IFN-γ and IL-12 cytokines when compared to M2 macrophages [123]. RANKL induces the differentiation of BMMs into M1 macrophages, which, in turn, targets M2 macrophage-specific factors OPN and RUNX2 for bone regeneration [124]. Subsequent research has indicated that IL-4 and IL-13 can elevate the proportion of M2 macrophages, leading to substantial improvement in bone regeneration during the ossification phase [125]. In contrast, experiments have been performed with OVX osteoporotic mice in the absence of estrogen. This experiment reveals that RANKL actively stimulates the differentiation of M2 macrophages into osteoclasts. This also indicates the protective role of estrogen over M2 macrophages against RANKL stimulation [126]. Collectively, these investigations highlight the significance of the plasticity and diversity of macrophages, positioning them as vital contributors to the preservation of bone homeostasis.

5.3 Dendritic cells

A surface covered with MHC-II and characterized by professional antigen-presenting cells serves as a link connecting the adaptive and innate immune responses. Recent emerging data proposes that dendritic cells (DCs) stimulate inflammation-driven osteoclastogenesis and amplify bone loss by serving as precursors to OCs, which have been supported by the whole genome sequencing data [127]. Both OCs and DCs exhibit the RANK receptor on their surfaces. This receptor not only facilitates DC interactions with T cells but also triggers the initiation of the NF-κB developmental signaling pathway, ultimately culminating in the process of osteoclastogenesis [128]. Under *in vitro* condition, DCs undergo trans-differentiation into OCs when exposed to M-CSF and RANKL. It has been noted that in comparison to OCs derived from monocytes, OC generation and fusion from DCs occur at a quicker pace [129]. However, a recent study has documented that interferon-λ1 (IFN-λ1) derived from DCs hinders the differentiation of osteoclasts by obstructing the NF-κB signaling pathway and the formation of the NLRP3 inflammasome. Moreover, the introduction of the IFN-λ1 monoclonal antibody was shown to reverse this impact [21]. DCs experience an extension of their lifespan and display increased levels of the cytokines IL-7 and IL-15 in conditions characterized by a lack of estrogen. Synchronized action of these cytokines triggers the production of pro-inflammatory cytokines IL-17A and TNF-α by T cells in antigen-independent way. These pro-inflammatory cytokines elicit the bone lesions in osteoporotic circumstances. This suggests the indirect influence of DCs in influencing bone health during estrogen deficiency [130]. T cell regulation influences the trans-differentiation process from DCs to OCs by controlling the secretion of IFN-γ. This interferon obstructs TRAF6, thereby hindering RANKL signaling. This obstruction leads to the inhibition of osteoclast maturation and activation [131]. Additionally, investigations also suggest that Th17 cells also play a role in governing the transformation from DCs to OCs. Moreover, under certain conditions, DCs have been observed to produce the anti-osteoporotic cytokine TGF-β [132]. To sum up, these studies indicate that dendritic cells perform a remarkable role in the regulation of osteoclastogenesis.

5.4 B cells

Following antigen stimulation, B cells undergo proliferation and differentiation into plasma cells. Emerging studies have implicated the role of B cells in regulation of the RANKL/OPG axis. This study has also revealed that B cells are one of the major sources of RANKL, which exacerbates bone loss in cases of ovariectomy-induced bone loss [133]. RA mice model study reveals that B cells directly suppress OBs differentiation by triggering the expression of OB inhibitors, such as CCL3 and TNF through ERK and NF-κB signaling pathways [134]. Moreover, another study revealed that RANKL stimulates B cell proliferation and subsequently function as supportive cells for osteoclasts [135]. In an inflammatory setting, activated T cells interact with B cells through the CD40/CD40L signaling pathway and stimulate OPG production, exerting a beneficial impact on the regeneration of bone tissue [136]. Additionally, TGF-β stimulates B cells to generate OPG, implying that B cells impede the process of osteoclast differentiation [137]. Recently, another subset of B cells, known as immunosuppressive B regulatory cells (Bregs) have been discovered. These cells have been shown to play immense role in the bone remodeling process [138]. The Bregs majorly produce IL-10 and IL-35. One study co-related the suppressed IL-10 levels along with low number of Bregs in osteoporotic mice model [139]. Additionally, IL-35 produced by these Bregs not only helps in B cell differentiation but also represses bone degeneration via induction of OPG along with suppressing RANKL production [139]. To conclude, the involvement of B cells in bone regeneration remains a subject of debate, and their precise function might be contingent on the specific pathological conditions present locally.

5.5 T cells

Originated from hematopoietic stem cells and matured at the thymus, T cells play immunoregulatory role through the production of various types of cytokines. While in the resting state, T cells can restrain bone resorption by osteoclasts. However, upon activation and the expression of RANKL, they participate in the creation of OCs, consequently amplifying bone resorption [131]. IFN-γ establishes an inverse relationship between T cell activation and the process of bone resorption. This is achieved as

IFN-γ intervenes with RANKL-RANK signaling and triggers the degradation of the RANK adaptor protein, specifically TRAF6. TRAF6 acts as an intermediary protein that instigates the survival and differentiation of osteoclasts by activating downstream signaling pathways through the interaction of RANKL and RANK [131]. T cells are classified into two primary subclasses: CD8+ T cells and CD4+ T cells. Within this group, CD4+ T cells encompass diverse subsets that perform a dual function: ensuring immune protection and participating in bone remodeling.

CD8+ T cells are well known for their cytotoxic activity against invading pathogens. CD8+ T cells also play protective role in bone remodeling process by profoundly suppressing osteoclastogenesis. Studies have revealed that CD8+ T cells do not exert a regulatory effect on osteoblastogenesis in an OPG-dependent manner, as evidenced by the fact that treatment with OPG does not result in any alteration of outcomes [140]. Administration of anabolic PTH treatment to mice is observed to notably elevate the synthesis of Wnt10b by CD8+ T cells found in the bone marrow. This, in turn, triggers the activation of canonical Wnt signaling within pre-osteoblasts. This finding underscores the pivotal role of T cells in the mechanism of anabolic PTH's effects [141]. Mice devoid of T cells display reduced Wnt signaling in pre-osteoblasts, resulting in compromised osteoblastic commitment, proliferation, differentiation, and lifespan. These collective effects ultimately lead to an attenuated anabolic response within trabecular bone and an inability to enhance bone strength [142].

CD4+ T cells regulate their immune-regulatory effect through cytokines secretion. It comprises various subsets, including Th1, Th2, Th9, Th17, TFh, and Th22 cells. IL-4 impedes osteoclastogenesis by suppressing the NFATc1 factor responsible for osteoclast differentiation. Furthermore, IL-4 hinders bone resorption by obstructing NF-κB and Ca^{2+} signaling in mature osteoclasts [143]. IFN-γ possesses the ability to directly inhibit osteoclastogenesis; however, it can also stimulate the generation of osteoclasts by inducing the expression of RANKL on activated T cells. Furthermore, the direct impact of IFN-γ on osteoclastogenesis varies depending on the stage of osteoclast differentiation [144]. RORγt-expressing Th17 cells play stimulating role in osteoclastogenesis primarily by generating IL-17. This cytokine acts on osteoclast precursors to stimulate RANK production, and it also induces the expression of RANKL in stromal cells and osteoblasts [145]. *In vitro* study has also revealed that Treg cells directly enhance the functionality of osteoblasts and enhance the osteogenic differentiation capacity of osteoblast precursor cells, such as bone marrow mesenchymal stem cells (BMMSCs) [146]. Additional investigations have demonstrated that Treg cells interact with CD8+ T cells to increase the production of WNT10b, which exerts its effects on stromal cells and osteoblasts, thereby promoting bone formation [147]. Th9 cells, characterized by the expression of PU.1, release IL-9, which influences the expression of various genes related to osteoclastogenesis, including matrix metalloproteinases (MMPs) [148]. IL-9 secretion substantially amplifies the differentiation of osteoclasts. A study noted that Th22 cells contribute to the differentiation of osteoclasts by releasing the IL-22 cytokine. This cytokine triggers the expression of NFATc1 in CD14+ monocytes, leading to exacerbated bone degradation in patients with rheumatoid arthritis (RA) [108]. Moreover, another study implies that IL-22, by increasing the expression of RANKL, prompts the differentiation of osteoclasts and induces bone resorption in the subchondral bone of temporomandibular joint osteoarthritis (TMJ-OA) and in cases of periodontitis [149]. To conclude, through several subsets, T cells play pivotal role in bone remodeling process.

6. Epigenetics of bone remodeling

Epigenetic regulation involves heritable changes in the DNA or gene loci to alter their expression pattern without any modification in the sequence of the corresponding DNA segments. Epigenetic modifications are essential in establishing cell fates, genomic imprinting, and differentiation of a particular cell type from their respective precursors. Any abnormality in such control mechanisms severely affects the cells and gives rise to various diseases including, autoimmune, somatic, metabolic, and even malignant tumors leading to cancer [150]. Recruitment and differentiation of these cells involve several growth factors and secreted cytokines, which induce several intracellular pathways and interaction of several transcription factors. Bone remodeling being such a critical process, is very tightly controlled by such epigenetic regulatory mechanisms [150]. In recent times, much-needed research has highlighted the importance of epigenetic regulatory mechanisms involved in bone remodeling. Studies delineating the roles of these genomic changes have garnered a lot of traction, and it has been shown that the differentiation of OBs and OCs is significantly dependent on epigenetic regulatory mechanisms [150]. Epigenetic alterations can be broadly classified into DNA modifications, histone modifications, chromatin remodeling, and transcription of noncoding RNAs. Methylation and hydroxy methylation of DNA are well known for repressing certain gene loci [151]. In contrast, histone tail modifications including acetylation, phosphorylation, ubiquitination, ribosylation, etc. critically regulate expression of a wide array of genes by both activating and repressing them [152] along with aiding in DNA repair. Chromatin-remodelers constitute three fundamental classes of proteins namely, readers, writers, and erasers. These proteins act in unison to control the expression pattern of a large variety of transcription factors, which, in turn, regulate the fates of the involved cells [153]. Detailing each of these processes is not possible within the finite limits of this chapter. Hence, the following sections will primarily focus on summarizing the augmentations of histone proteins and their modulation of bone remodeling.

6.1 Histone modifications

Histones constitute a class of small proteins that provide structural support to chromosomes and help in compacting the genomic material in a eukaryotic cell. The histone proteins are also responsible for regulating the expression of genes by harboring several marks called histone modifications. This enables the modified histone proteins to directly interfere with the compaction of chromatin and recruit other protein complexes to alter their target gene transcription. Modifications involve addition of specific chemical groups to exposed residues on the N-terminal tails of these histones.

6.1.1 Histone acetylation

Acetylation of histone tails primarily occurs at the ε-amino group of the lysine residues. This transfer reaction is catalyzed by histone acetyltransferases or HATs. Acetylation of histones results in the opening of the chromatin due to removal of positive charges from the histone tail and making the regulatory regions more accessible to the TF complexes, which generally act as gene activation marks. They can also serve as DNA repair signals. Several studies have indicated that class I HATs, such as p300/CBP, are recruited to the promoters of numerous pro-osteoblastic genes, such as RUNX2, and OSX among others [154, 155]. In one such study, Kim et al. observed that the vitamin D receptor facilitated the recruitment of CBP and p300 to the promoters of CYP and OPN genes during exposure to 1, 25-dihydroxyvitamin D3 [155]. This recruitment subsequently results in the enhanced acetylation of histone H4 in osteoblasts. p300/CBP-associated factor (PCAF/KAT2B) is an additional histone acetyltransferase (HAT) that plays a crucial role in the process of osteogenic differentiation [155]. PCAF expression gets upregulated following osteogenic induction mediated by Smad signaling resulting in an increased expression of BMP pathway genes through the augmentation of histone H3K9 acetylation [154]. Recent genome-wide association studies have examined the chromatin landscape during the process of osteogenesis from MSCs, which display a significant increase in the levels of H3K9Ac, H4K5Ac, and H3K27Ac marks globally [156]. Similar to osteoblast differentiation, osteoclastogenesis is also influenced by histone acetylation. One study indicates that targeted pharmacological suppression of Bromodomain and PHD finger-containing protein significantly hinders the process of RANKL-induced differentiation, namely in the formation of osteoclasts responsible for bone resorption [157].

HDACs also control the epigenetic landscape by reversing the effects of acetylation. Evidently, the expression of osteoblast-related genes is decreased by HDAC1, HDAC2, HDAC3, and HDAC8 [158]. HDAC1 is indeed recruited to the promoter regions of OSX and OCN, leading to the suppression of osteoblast development [159]. Similarly, HDAC3 and RUNX2 are found to interact and result in the repression of the OCN promoter, leading to the subsequent inhibition of osteoblast development [160]. HDAC3 is also found to control the expression of important osteogenic factors, such as RUNX2 and Col1a [160]. Sirtuin 1 (SIRT1) (another class of HDACs), has been found to enhance the differentiation of BMSCs into osteoblasts. Moreover, SIRT1 can facilitate the deacetylation of β-catenin, disrupting the Wnt/β-catenin pathway and resulting in its increased localization within the nucleus and upregulate osteoblast function [47].

6.1.2 Histone methylation

Methylation of histone takes place on several basic residues, including lysine, histidine, and arginine. Major methylation marks can be found on various H3 and H4 residues, including H3K4, H3K9, H3R17, H3K79, H4R3, H4K20, and H4K59. Methylation marks on histones can act as both transcriptional activators (H3K4, H3K79, H3K36, and H3R17), and silencers (H3K9, H3K27, and H3K20). Similar to what is observed during histone acetylation, methylation of histones is also carried out by histone methyl transferases or HMTs. Studies have found that H3K36 tri-methylation increases the interaction of RUNX2 and p300, leading to upregulation of osteogenic genes [158]. Recent studies have revealed interesting insights about additional histone methylation marks that can control the osteoblastic differentiation form BDMSCs. Levels of H3K4me3 and H3K36me3 are found to be increased significantly on a global scale [161]. Corresponding decrease on repressive methylation marks, such as H3K27me3, is also evident [161]. The essentiality of multipotent development of MSCs has been determined through the identification of active histone marks, including, H3K4me1, H3K4me3, and H3K36me3 during osteoblastic differentiation [156]. Another important HMT, EZH2 is shown to promote H3K27 tri-methylation of the promoters of key regulatory genes such as RUNX2, OPN, OSC, MX1, FHL-1, etc. and suppress osteoclastogenesis [162]. Similarly, PRMT5 (another methyl transferase) is found to suppress osteoblastic differentiation [163]. It is responsible for the global methylation of arginine residues on H3R8 and H4R3. Blocking this symmetric demethylation enhances osteogenic differentiation of MSCs, indicating the importance of PRMT5 activity on fate specification of MSCs during osteogenesis [163]. During osteoclastogenesis, EZH2 is found to positively boost the osteoclast activity by downregulating IRF8 (a known negative regulator). The IRF8 gene promoter has increased repressive H3K27me3 marks *via* recruitment of EZH2 by RANKL [164]. In contrast, DOT1L methyl transferase is found to suppress osteoclast formation by methylating H3K79 [165].

Just as HMTs, histone demethylases are crucial in maintaining the right balance to control the important cell specification fates. Enzymes like JMJD3 (KDM6B) demethylate H3K27 to upregulate key genes, such as RUNX2, OCX, OSN, etc. to boost osteoblast differentiation [166]. Interestingly, JMJD3 also endorses osteoclast formation by upregulating NFATC1 gene in T-cells *via* restricting repressive histone marks at its promoter [167]. Another demethylase, JARID1B, was shown to demethylate RUNX2 promoter leading to suppressed osteoblastic lineage specification [168]. Thus, the critical balance between histone methylation and demethylation controls the lineage specification of both OBs and OCs to ensure smoother osteogenic turnover.

7. Conclusion

In addition to providing structural support and protecting interior organs, bones also play a number of metabolic roles, particularly in preserving the body's mineral balance. When bone resorption outpaces bone creation, bone loss will take place and, in extreme situations, result in osteoporosis. The pathophysiology of aberrant bone metabolism and osteoporosis will be better understood *via* a thorough investigation of these epigenetic pathways. However, very little is now known about the epigenetics of anomalies in bone remodeling. Further, research is needed to understand the known epigenetic regulatory factors, mechanisms, and the connection between their downstream target genes and associated disorders. The mechanisms of epigenetic modification and histone alterations also need to be clarified. The clinical diagnosis and management of osteoporosis will be greatly enhanced by the discovery of specific biomarkers connected to the condition. A comprehensive epigenetic spectrum of healthy bone and bone illnesses based on the entire genome will be established thanks to the widespread application of epigenetic microarrays, high-throughput sequencing, and other emerging technologies. The biological underpinnings of the fundamental molecular mechanisms of bone remodeling and the delicate balance between anabolism and catabolism in bone tissue will be further revealed by additional study in this field, opening up new avenues for the diagnosis and treatment of common bone remodeling disorders.

Acknowledgements

The authors acknowledge Mr. Biswajit Biswas for his invaluable insights in preparing the figures.

The authors also acknowledge the funding from SERB (CRG/2019/001049).

Conflict of interest

The authors declare no conflict of interest.

Author details

Sayantee Hazra†, Shagnik Chattopadhyay† and Ritobrata Goswami*
School of Bioscience, IIT Kharagpur, India

*Address all correspondence to: ritobrata@gmail.com

† These authors contributed equally.

References

[1] Okamoto K, Nakashima T, Shinohara M, Negishi-Koga T, Komatsu N, Terashima A, et al. Osteoimmunology: The conceptual framework unifying the immune and skeletal systems. Physiological Reviews. 2017;**97**(4):1295-1349

[2] Kenkre JS, Bassett J. The bone remodelling cycle. Annals of Clinical Biochemistry. 2018;**55**(3):308-327

[3] Loi F, Cordova LA, Pajarinen J, Lin TH, Yao Z, Goodman SB. Inflammation, fracture and bone repair. Bone. 2016;**86**:119-130

[4] Feng X, McDonald JM. Disorders of bone remodeling. Annual Review of Pathology. 2011;**6**:121-145

[5] Rowe P, Koller A, Sharma S. Physiology, bone remodeling. In: StatPearls. Treasure Island (FL): StatPearls Publishing; 2023

[6] Bonucci E, Ballanti P. Osteoporosis-bone remodeling and animal models. Toxicologic Pathology. 2014;**42**(6):957-969

[7] Feng X. Chemical and biochemical basis of cell-bone matrix interaction in health and disease. Current Chemical Biology. 2009;**3**(2):189-196

[8] Marion NW, Mao JJ. Mesenchymal stem cells and tissue engineering. Methods in Enzymology. 2006;**420**:339-361

[9] Zhao E, Xu H, Wang L, Kryczek I, Wu K, Hu Y, et al. Bone marrow and the control of immunity. Cellular & Molecular Immunology. 2012;**9**(1):11-19

[10] Sozen T, Ozisik L, Basaran NC. An overview and management of osteoporosis. European Journal of Rheumatology. 2017;**4**(1):46-56

[11] Srivastava RK, Dar HY, Mishra PK. Immunoporosis: Immunology of osteoporosis-role of T cells. Frontiers in Immunology. 2018;**9**:657

[12] Saxena Y, Routh S, Mukhopadhaya A. Immunoporosis: Role of innate immune cells in osteoporosis. Frontiers in Immunology. 2021;**12**:687037

[13] Singh K, Piprode V, Mhaske ST, Barhanpurkar-Naik A, Wani MR. IL-3 differentially regulates membrane and soluble RANKL in osteoblasts through metalloproteases and the JAK2/STAT5 pathway and improves the RANKL/OPG ratio in adult mice. Journal of Immunology. 2018;**200**(2):595-606

[14] Abu-Amer Y. IL-4 abrogates osteoclastogenesis through STAT6-dependent inhibition of NF-kappaB. The Journal of Clinical Investigation. 2001;**107**(11):1375-1385

[15] Moore KW, de Waal MR, Coffman RL, O'Garra A. Interleukin-10 and the interleukin-10 receptor. Annual Review of Immunology. 2001;**19**:683-765

[16] Nagata N, Kitaura H, Yoshida N, Nakayama K. Inhibition of RANKL-induced osteoclast formation in mouse bone marrow cells by IL-12: Involvement of IFN-gamma possibly induced from non-T cell population. Bone. 2003;**33**(4):721-732

[17] Stein NC, Kreutzmann C, Zimmermann SP, Niebergall U, Hellmeyer L, Goettsch C, et al. Interleukin-4 and interleukin-13 stimulate the osteoclast inhibitor

osteoprotegerin by human endothelial cells through the STAT6 pathway. Journal of Bone and Mineral Research. 2008;**23**(5):750-758

[18] Kitaura H, Fujimura Y, Yoshimatsu M, Kohara H, Morita Y, Aonuma T, et al. IL-12- and IL-18-mediated, nitric oxide-induced apoptosis in TNF-alpha-mediated osteoclastogenesis of bone marrow cells. Calcified Tissue International. 2011; **89**(1):65-73

[19] Tsubaki M, Takeda T, Matsuda T, Yamamoto Y, Higashinaka A, Yamamoto K, et al. Interleukin 19 suppresses RANKL-induced osteoclastogenesis via the inhibition of NF-kappaB and p38MAPK activation and c-Fos expression in RAW264.7 cells. Cytokine. 2021;**144**:155591

[20] Furukawa M, Takaishi H, Takito J, Yoda M, Sakai S, Hikata T, et al. IL-27 abrogates receptor activator of NF-kappa B ligand-mediated osteoclastogenesis of human granulocyte-macrophage colony-forming unit cells through STAT1-dependent inhibition of c-Fos. Journal of Immunology. 2009;**183**(4):2397-2406

[21] Chen Y, Wang Y, Tang R, Yang J, Dou C, Dong Y, et al. Dendritic cells-derived interferon-lambda1 ameliorated inflammatory bone destruction through inhibiting osteoclastogenesis. Cell Death & Disease. 2020;**11**(6):414

[22] Yan H, Dong M, Liu X, Shen Q, He D, Huang X, et al. Multiple myeloma cell-derived IL-32gamma increases the immunosuppressive function of macrophages by promoting indoleamine 2,3-dioxygenase (IDO) expression. Cancer Letters. 2019;**446**:38-48

[23] Lima IL, Macari S, Madeira MF, Rodrigues LF, Colavite PM, Garlet GP, et al. Osteoprotective effects of IL-33/ST2 link to osteoclast apoptosis. The American Journal of Pathology. 2015; **185**(12):3338-3348

[24] Peng M, Wang Y, Qiang L, Xu Y, Li C, Li T, et al. Interleukin-35 inhibits TNF-alpha-induced osteoclastogenesis and promotes apoptosis via shifting the activation from TNF receptor-associated death domain (TRADD)-TRAF2 to TRADD-Fas-associated death domain by JAK1/STAT1. Frontiers in Immunology. 2018;**9**:1417

[25] Takayanagi H, Sato K, Takaoka A, Taniguchi T. Interplay between interferon and other cytokine systems in bone metabolism. Immunological Reviews. 2005;**208**:181-193

[26] Sims NA, Jenkins BJ, Nakamura A, Quinn JM, Li R, Gillespie MT, et al. Interleukin-11 receptor signaling is required for normal bone remodeling. Journal of Bone and Mineral Research. 2005;**20**(7):1093-1102

[27] Kim JH, Jin HM, Kim K, Song I, Youn BU, Matsuo K, et al. The mechanism of osteoclast differentiation induced by IL-1. Journal of Immunology. 2009;**183**(3):1862-1870

[28] Rose-John S. Interleukin-6 family cytokines. Cold Spring Harbor Perspectives in Biology. 2018;**10**(2):a028415

[29] Toraldo G, Roggia C, Qian WP, Pacifici R, Weitzmann MN. IL-7 induces bone loss in vivo by induction of receptor activator of nuclear factor kappa B ligand and tumor necrosis factor alpha from T cells. Proceedings of the National Academy of Sciences of the United States of America. 2003;**100**(1): 125-130

[30] Kopesky P, Tiedemann K, Alkekhia D, Zechner C, Millard B,

Schoeberl B, et al. Autocrine signaling is a key regulatory element during osteoclastogenesis. Biology Open. 2014; **3**(8):767-776

[31] Okabe I, Kikuchi T, Mogi M, Takeda H, Aino M, Kamiya Y, et al. IL-15 and RANKL play a synergistically important role in osteoclastogenesis. Journal of Cellular Biochemistry. 2017; **118**(4):739-747

[32] Tyagi AM, Srivastava K, Mansoori MN, Trivedi R, Chattopadhyay N, Singh D. Estrogen deficiency induces the differentiation of IL-17 secreting Th17 cells: A new candidate in the pathogenesis of osteoporosis. PLoS One. 2012;**7**(9): e44552

[33] Hsu YH, Chen WY, Chan CH, Wu CH, Sun ZJ, Chang MS. Anti-IL-20 monoclonal antibody inhibits the differentiation of osteoclasts and protects against osteoporotic bone loss. The Journal of Experimental Medicine. 2011;**208**(9):1849-1861

[34] Cheng X, Wan QL, Li ZB. AG490 suppresses interleukin-34-mediated osteoclastogenesis in mice bone marrow macrophages. Cell Biology International. 2017;**41**(6):659-668

[35] Chen L, Wei XQ, Evans B, Jiang W, Aeschlimann D. IL-23 promotes osteoclast formation by up-regulation of receptor activator of NF-kappaB (RANK) expression in myeloid precursor cells. European Journal of Immunology. 2008;**38**(10): 2845-2854

[36] Khapli SM, Mangashetti LS, Yogesha SD, Wani MR. IL-3 acts directly on osteoclast precursors and irreversibly inhibits receptor activator of NF-kappa B ligand-induced osteoclast differentiation by diverting the cells to macrophage lineage. Journal of Immunology. 2003; **171**(1):142-151

[37] Yogesha SD, Khapli SM, Wani MR. Interleukin-3 and granulocyte-macrophage colony-stimulating factor inhibits tumor necrosis factor (TNF)-alpha-induced osteoclast differentiation by down-regulation of expression of TNF receptors 1 and 2. The Journal of Biological Chemistry. 2005; **280**(12):11759-11769

[38] Yogesha SD, Khapli SM, Srivastava RK, Mangashetti LS, Pote ST, Mishra GC, et al. IL-3 inhibits TNF-alpha-induced bone resorption and prevents inflammatory arthritis. Journal of Immunology. 2009;**182**(1):361-370

[39] Oh J, Lee MS, Yeon JT, Choi SW, Kim HS, Shim H, et al. Inhibitory regulation of osteoclast differentiation by interleukin-3 via regulation of c-Fos and Id protein expression. Journal of Cellular Physiology. 2012;**227**(5): 1851-1860

[40] Gupta N, Barhanpurkar AP, Tomar GB, Srivastava RK, Kour S, Pote ST, et al. IL-3 inhibits human osteoclastogenesis and bone resorption through downregulation of c-Fms and diverts the cells to dendritic cell lineage. Journal of Immunology. 2010;**185**(4): 2261-2272

[41] Lee J, Seong S, Kim JH, Kim K, Kim I, Jeong BC, et al. STAT5 is a key transcription factor for IL-3-mediated inhibition of RANKL-induced osteoclastogenesis. Scientific Reports. 2016;**6**:30977

[42] Barhanpurkar AP, Gupta N, Srivastava RK, Tomar GB, Naik SP, Joshi SR, et al. IL-3 promotes osteoblast differentiation and bone formation in human mesenchymal stem cells.

Biochemical and Biophysical Research Communications. 2012;**418**(4):669-675

[43] Wei S, Wang MW, Teitelbaum SL, Ross FP. Interleukin-4 reversibly inhibits osteoclastogenesis via inhibition of NF-kappa B and mitogen-activated protein kinase signaling. The Journal of Biological Chemistry. 2002;**277**(8):6622-6630

[44] Cheng J, Liu J, Shi Z, Xu D, Luo S, Siegal GP, et al. Interleukin-4 inhibits RANKL-induced NFATc1 expression via STAT6: A novel mechanism mediating its blockade of osteoclastogenesis. Journal of Cellular Biochemistry. 2011; **112**(11):3385-3392

[45] te Velde AA, Huijbens RJ, Heije K, de Vries JE, Figdor CG. Interleukin-4 (IL-4) inhibits secretion of IL-1 beta, tumor necrosis factor alpha, and IL-6 by human monocytes. Blood. 1990;**76**(7): 1392-1397

[46] Hiasa M, Abe M, Nakano A, Oda A, Amou H, Kido S, et al. GM-CSF and IL-4 induce dendritic cell differentiation and disrupt osteoclastogenesis through M-CSF receptor shedding by up-regulation of TNF-alpha converting enzyme (TACE). Blood. 2009;**114**(20):4517-4526

[47] Liu D, Yao S, Wise GE. Effect of interleukin-10 on gene expression of osteoclastogenic regulatory molecules in the rat dental follicle. European Journal of Oral Sciences. 2006;**114**(1):42-49

[48] Park-Min KH, Ji JD, Antoniv T, Reid AC, Silver RB, Humphrey MB, et al. IL-10 suppresses calcium-mediated costimulation of receptor activator NF-kappa B signaling during human osteoclast differentiation by inhibiting TREM-2 expression. Journal of Immunology. 2009;**183**(4):2444-2455

[49] Mohamed SG, Sugiyama E, Shinoda K, Taki H, Hounoki H, Abdel-Aziz HO, et al. Interleukin-10 inhibits RANKL-mediated expression of NFATc1 in part via suppression of c-Fos and c-Jun in RAW264.7 cells and mouse bone marrow cells. Bone. 2007;**41**(4): 592-602

[50] Ma X, Zhu X, He X, Yi X, Jin A. The Wnt pathway regulator expression levels and their relationship to bone metabolism in thoracolumbar osteoporotic vertebral compression fracture patients. American Journal of Translational Research. 2021;**13**(5): 4812-4818

[51] Dresner-Pollak R, Gelb N, Rachmilewitz D, Karmeli F, Weinreb M. Interleukin 10-deficient mice develop osteopenia, decreased bone formation, and mechanical fragility of long bones. Gastroenterology. 2004;**127**(3):792-801

[52] de Waal MR, Abrams J, Bennett B, Figdor CG, de Vries JE. Interleukin 10 (IL-10) inhibits cytokine synthesis by human monocytes: An autoregulatory role of IL-10 produced by monocytes. The Journal of Experimental Medicine. 1991;**174**(5):1209-1220

[53] Kawashima I, Ohsumi J, Mita-Honjo K, Shimoda-Takano K, Ishikawa H, Sakakibara S, et al. Molecular cloning of cDNA encoding adipogenesis inhibitory factor and identity with interleukin-11. FEBS Letters. 1991;**283**(2):199-202

[54] Kudo O, Sabokbar A, Pocock A, Itonaga I, Fujikawa Y, Athanasou NA. Interleukin-6 and interleukin-11 support human osteoclast formation by a RANKL-independent mechanism. Bone. 2003;**32**(1):1-7

[55] Takeuchi Y, Watanabe S, Ishii G, Takeda S, Nakayama K, Fukumoto S, et al. Interleukin-11 as a stimulatory factor for bone formation prevents bone loss with advancing age in mice. The

Journal of Biological Chemistry. 2002; **277**(50):49011-49018

[56] Hsu YH, Hsieh PP, Chang MS. Interleukin-19 blockade attenuates collagen-induced arthritis in rats. Rheumatology (Oxford, England). 2012; **51**(3):434-442

[57] Amcheslavsky A, Bar-Shavit Z. Interleukin (IL)-12 mediates the anti-osteoclastogenic activity of CpG-oligodeoxynucleotides. Journal of Cellular Physiology. 2006;**207**(1): 244-250

[58] Udagawa N, Horwood NJ, Elliott J, Mackay A, Owens J, Okamura H, et al. Interleukin-18 (interferon-gamma-inducing factor) is produced by osteoblasts and acts via granulocyte/macrophage colony-stimulating factor and not via interferon-gamma to inhibit osteoclast formation. The Journal of Experimental Medicine. 1997;**185**(6): 1005-1012

[59] Mansoori MN, Shukla P, Kakaji M, Tyagi AM, Srivastava K, Shukla M, et al. IL-18BP is decreased in osteoporotic women: Prevents inflammasome mediated IL-18 activation and reduces Th17 differentiation. Scientific Reports. 2016;**6**:33680

[60] Onoe Y, Miyaura C, Kaminakayashiki T, Nagai Y, Noguchi K, Chen QR, et al. IL-13 and IL-4 inhibit bone resorption by suppressing cyclooxygenase-2-dependent prostaglandin synthesis in osteoblasts. Journal of Immunology. 1996;**156**(2): 758-764

[61] Kalliolias GD, Zhao B, Triantafyllopoulou A, Park-Min KH, Ivashkiv LB. Interleukin-27 inhibits human osteoclastogenesis by abrogating RANKL-mediated induction of nuclear factor of activated T cells c1 and suppressing proximal RANK signaling. Arthritis and Rheumatism. 2010;**62**(2): 402-413

[62] Shukla P, Mansoori MN, Kakaji M, Shukla M, Gupta SK, Singh D. Interleukin 27 (IL-27) alleviates bone loss in estrogen-deficient conditions by induction of early growth response-2 gene. The Journal of Biological Chemistry. 2017;**292**(11):4686-4699

[63] Peng Q, Luo A, Zhou Z, Xuan W, Qiu M, Wu Q, et al. Interleukin 29 inhibits RANKL-induced osteoclastogenesis via activation of JNK and STAT, and inhibition of NF-kappaB and NFATc1. Cytokine. 2019;**113**: 144-154

[64] Kiyomiya H, Ariyoshi W, Okinaga T, Kaneuji T, Mitsugi S, Sakurai T, et al. IL-33 inhibits RANKL-induced osteoclast formation through the regulation of Blimp-1 and IRF-8 expression. Biochemical and Biophysical Research Communications. 2015;**460**(2): 320-326

[65] Saleh H, Eeles D, Hodge JM, Nicholson GC, Gu R, Pompolo S, et al. Interleukin-33, a target of parathyroid hormone and oncostatin m, increases osteoblastic matrix mineral deposition and inhibits osteoclast formation in vitro. Endocrinology. 2011;**152**(5): 1911-1922

[66] De Martinis M, Ginaldi L, Sirufo MM, Bassino EM, De Pietro F, Pioggia G, et al. IL-33/vitamin D crosstalk in psoriasis-associated osteoporosis. Frontiers in Immunology. 2020;**11**:604055

[67] Ohori F, Kitaura H, Ogawa S, Shen WR, Qi J, Noguchi T, et al. IL-33 inhibits TNF-alpha-induced Osteoclastogenesis and bone resorption.

International Journal of Molecular Sciences. 2020;**21**(3):1130

[68] Schulze J, Bickert T, Beil FT, Zaiss MM, Albers J, Wintges K, et al. Interleukin-33 is expressed in differentiated osteoblasts and blocks osteoclast formation from bone marrow precursor cells. Journal of Bone and Mineral Research. 2011;**26**(4):704-717

[69] Ginaldi L, De Martinis M, Saitta S, Sirufo MM, Mannucci C, Casciaro M, et al. Interleukin-33 serum levels in postmenopausal women with osteoporosis. Scientific Reports. 2019; **9**(1):3786

[70] Zhang H, Li Y, Yuan L, Yao L, Yang J, Xia L, et al. Interleukin-35 is involved in angiogenesis/bone remodeling coupling through T helper 17/Interleukin-17 Axis. Frontiers in Endocrinology. 2021;**12**:642676

[71] Li Y, Wang X, Lu J. Interleukin-35 promote osteogenesis and inhibit adipogenesis: Role of Wnt/beta-catenin and PPARgamma signaling pathways. Inflammation. 2023;**46**(2):522-533

[72] Mun SH, Ko NY, Kim HS, Kim JW, Kim DK, Kim AR, et al. Interleukin-33 stimulates formation of functional osteoclasts from human CD14(+) monocytes. Cellular and Molecular Life Sciences. 2010;**67**(22):3883-3892

[73] Kobayashi K, Takahashi N, Jimi E, Udagawa N, Takami M, Kotake S, et al. Tumor necrosis factor alpha stimulates osteoclast differentiation by a mechanism independent of the ODF/RANKL-RANK interaction. The Journal of Experimental Medicine. 2000; **191**(2):275-286

[74] Yamashita T, Yao Z, Li F, Zhang Q, Badell IR, Schwarz EM, et al. NF-kappaB p50 and p52 regulate receptor activator of NF-kappaB ligand (RANKL) and tumor necrosis factor-induced osteoclast precursor differentiation by activating c-Fos and NFATc1. The Journal of Biological Chemistry. 2007;**282**(25): 18245-18253

[75] Matsuo K, Galson DL, Zhao C, Peng L, Laplace C, Wang KZ, et al. Nuclear factor of activated T-cells (NFAT) rescues osteoclastogenesis in precursors lacking c-Fos. The Journal of Biological Chemistry. 2004;**279**(25): 26475-26480

[76] Yao Z, Xing L, Qin C, Schwarz EM, Boyce BF. Osteoclast precursor interaction with bone matrix induces osteoclast formation directly by an interleukin-1-mediated autocrine mechanism. The Journal of Biological Chemistry. 2008;**283**(15):9917-9924

[77] Mizukami J, Takaesu G, Akatsuka H, Sakurai H, Ninomiya-Tsuji J, Matsumoto K, et al. Receptor activator of NF-kappaB ligand (RANKL) activates TAK1 mitogen-activated protein kinase kinase kinase through a signaling complex containing RANK, TAB2, and TRAF6. Molecular and Cellular Biology. 2002;**22**(4):992-1000

[78] Yao Z, Lei W, Duan R, Li Y, Luo L, Boyce BF. RANKL cytokine enhances TNF-induced osteoclastogenesis independently of TNF receptor associated factor (TRAF) 6 by degrading TRAF3 in osteoclast precursors. The Journal of Biological Chemistry. 2017; **292**(24):10169-10179

[79] Gilbert L, He X, Farmer P, Boden S, Kozlowski M, Rubin J, et al. Inhibition of osteoblast differentiation by tumor necrosis factor-alpha. Endocrinology. 2000;**141**(11):3956-3964

[80] Polzer K, Joosten L, Gasser J, Distler JH, Ruiz G, Baum W, et al.

Interleukin-1 is essential for systemic inflammatory bone loss. Annals of the Rheumatic Diseases. 2010;**69**(1):284-290

[81] Wei S, Kitaura H, Zhou P, Ross FP, Teitelbaum SL. IL-1 mediates TNF-induced osteoclastogenesis. The Journal of Clinical Investigation. 2005;**115**(2): 282-290

[82] Tanabe N, Maeno M, Suzuki N, Fujisaki K, Tanaka H, Ogiso B, et al. IL-1 alpha stimulates the formation of osteoclast-like cells by increasing M-CSF and PGE2 production and decreasing OPG production by osteoblasts. Life Sciences. 2005;**77**(6):615-626

[83] Palmqvist P, Persson E, Conaway HH, Lerner UH. IL-6, leukemia inhibitory factor, and oncostatin M stimulate bone resorption and regulate the expression of receptor activator of NF-kappa B ligand, osteoprotegerin, and receptor activator of NF-kappa B in mouse calvariae. Journal of Immunology. 2002;**169**(6): 3353-3362

[84] De Benedetti F, Rucci N, Del Fattore A, Peruzzi B, Paro R, Longo M, et al. Impaired skeletal development in interleukin-6-transgenic mice: A model for the impact of chronic inflammation on the growing skeletal system. Arthritis and Rheumatism. 2006;**54**(11):3551-3563

[85] Lazzaro L, Tonkin BA, Poulton IJ, McGregor NE, Ferlin W, Sims NA. IL-6 trans-signalling mediates trabecular, but not cortical, bone loss after ovariectomy. Bone. 2018;**112**:120-127

[86] Liu H, Feng W, Yimin CJ, Lv S, Hasegawa T, et al. Histological evidence of increased osteoclast cell number and asymmetric bone resorption activity in the tibiae of Interleukin-6-deficient mice. The Journal of Histochemistry and Cytochemistry. 2014;**62**(8):556-564

[87] Yoshitake F, Itoh S, Narita H, Ishihara K, Ebisu S. Interleukin-6 directly inhibits osteoclast differentiation by suppressing receptor activator of NF-kappaB signaling pathways. The Journal of Biological Chemistry. 2008;**283**(17):11535-11540

[88] Feng W, Liu H, Luo T, Liu D, Du J, Sun J, et al. Combination of IL-6 and sIL-6R differentially regulate varying levels of RANKL-induced osteoclastogenesis through NF-kappaB, ERK and JNK signaling pathways. Scientific Reports. 2017;7:41411

[89] Zhu S, He H, Gao C, Luo G, Xie Y, Wang H, et al. Ovariectomy-induced bone loss in TNFalpha and IL6 gene knockout mice is regulated by different mechanisms. Journal of Molecular Endocrinology. 2018;**60**(3):185-198

[90] Li X, Zhou ZY, Zhang YY, Yang HL. IL-6 contributes to the defective osteogenesis of bone marrow stromal cells from the vertebral body of the glucocorticoid-induced osteoporotic mouse. PLoS One. 2016;**11**(4):e0154677

[91] Xie Z, Tang S, Ye G, Wang P, Li J, Liu W, et al. Interleukin-6/interleukin-6 receptor complex promotes osteogenic differentiation of bone marrow-derived mesenchymal stem cells. Stem Cell Research & Therapy. 2018;**9**(1):13

[92] Kaneshiro S, Ebina K, Shi K, Higuchi C, Hirao M, Okamoto M, et al. IL-6 negatively regulates osteoblast differentiation through the SHP2/MEK2 and SHP2/Akt2 pathways in vitro. Journal of Bone and Mineral Metabolism. 2014;**32**(4):378-392

[93] Salopek D, Grcevic D, Katavic V, Kovacic N, Lukic IK, Marusic A. Increased bone resorption and osteopenia are a part of the lymphoproliferative phenotype of mice

with systemic over-expression of interleukin-7 gene driven by MHC class II promoter. Immunology Letters. 2008; **121**(2):134-139

[94] Ryan MR, Shepherd R, Leavey JK, Gao Y, Grassi F, Schnell FJ, et al. An IL-7-dependent rebound in thymic T cell output contributes to the bone loss induced by estrogen deficiency. Proceedings of the National Academy of Sciences of the United States of America. 2005;**102**(46):16735-16740

[95] Miller JP, Izon D, DeMuth W, Gerstein R, Bhandoola A, Allman D. The earliest step in B lineage differentiation from common lymphoid progenitors is critically dependent upon interleukin 7. The Journal of Experimental Medicine. 2002;**196**(5):705-711

[96] Zhao JJ, Wu ZF, Yu YH, Wang L, Cheng L. Effects of interleukin-7/ interleukin-7 receptor on RANKL-mediated osteoclast differentiation and ovariectomy-induced bone loss by regulating c-Fos/c-Jun pathway. Journal of Cellular Physiology. 2018;**233**(9): 7182-7194

[97] Lee SK, Kalinowski JF, Jastrzebski SL, Puddington L, Lorenzo JA. Interleukin-7 is a direct inhibitor of in vitro osteoclastogenesis. Endocrinology. 2003;**144**(8): 3524-3531

[98] Takeda H, Kikuchi T, Soboku K, Okabe I, Mizutani H, Mitani A, et al. Effect of IL-15 and natural killer cells on osteoclasts and osteoblasts in a mouse coculture. Inflammation. 2014;**37**(3): 657-669

[99] Chen Z, Buki K, Vaaraniemi J, Gu G, Vaananen HK. The critical role of IL-34 in osteoclastogenesis. PLoS One. 2011; **6**(4):e18689

[100] Dixit M, Singh KB, Prakash R, Singh D. Functional block of IL-17 cytokine promotes bone healing by augmenting FOXO1 and ATF4 activity in cortical bone defect model. Osteoporosis International. 2017;**28**(7): 2207-2220

[101] Bhadricha H, Patel V, Singh AK, Savardekar L, Patil A, Surve S, et al. Increased frequency of Th17 cells and IL-17 levels are associated with low bone mineral density in postmenopausal women. Scientific Reports. 2021;**11**(1): 16155

[102] Lubberts E, van den Bersselaar L, Oppers-Walgreen B, Schwarzenberger P, Coenen-de Roo CJ, Kolls JK, et al. IL-17 promotes bone erosion in murine collagen-induced arthritis through loss of the receptor activator of NF-kappa B ligand/ osteoprotegerin balance. Journal of Immunology. 2003;**170**(5):2655-2662

[103] Kitami S, Tanaka H, Kawato T, Tanabe N, Katono-Tani T, Zhang F, et al. IL-17A suppresses the expression of bone resorption-related proteinases and osteoclast differentiation via IL-17RA or IL-17RC receptors in RAW264.7 cells. Biochimie. 2010;**92**(4):398-404

[104] Huang H, Kim HJ, Chang EJ, Lee ZH, Hwang SJ, Kim HM, et al. IL-17 stimulates the proliferation and differentiation of human mesenchymal stem cells: Implications for bone remodeling. Cell Death and Differentiation. 2009;**16**(10):1332-1343

[105] Wang Z, Tan J, Lei L, Sun W, Wu Y, Ding P, et al. The positive effects of secreting cytokines IL-17 and IFN-gamma on the early-stage differentiation and negative effects on the calcification of primary osteoblasts in vitro. International Immunopharmacology. 2018;**57**:1-10

[106] Lei L, Sun J, Han J, Jiang X, Wang Z, Chen L. Interleukin-17 induces pyroptosis in osteoblasts through the NLRP3 inflammasome pathway in vitro. International Immunopharmacology. 2021;**96**:107781

[107] Hsu YH, Chiu YS, Chen WY, Huang KY, Jou IM, Wu PT, et al. Anti-IL-20 monoclonal antibody promotes bone fracture healing through regulating IL-20-mediated osteoblastogenesis. Scientific Reports. 2016;**6**:24339

[108] Miyazaki Y, Nakayamada S, Kubo S, Nakano K, Iwata S, Miyagawa I, et al. Th22 cells promote osteoclast differentiation via production of IL-22 in rheumatoid arthritis. Frontiers in Immunology. 2018;**9**:2901

[109] Sato K, Suematsu A, Okamoto K, Yamaguchi A, Morishita Y, Kadono Y, et al. Th17 functions as an osteoclastogenic helper T cell subset that links T cell activation and bone destruction. The Journal of Experimental Medicine. 2006;**203**(12):2673-2682

[110] Quinn JM, Sims NA, Saleh H, Mirosa D, Thompson K, Bouralexis S, et al. IL-23 inhibits osteoclastogenesis indirectly through lymphocytes and is required for the maintenance of bone mass in mice. Journal of Immunology. 2008;**181**(8):5720-5729

[111] Nathan C. Neutrophils and immunity: Challenges and opportunities. Nature Reviews. Immunology. 2006; **6**(3):173-182

[112] Wagner C, Iking-Konert C, Denefleh B, Stegmaier S, Hug F, Hansch GM. Granzyme B and perforin: Constitutive expression in human polymorphonuclear neutrophils. Blood. 2004;**103**(3):1099-1104

[113] Bastian OW, Koenderman L, Alblas J, Leenen LP, Blokhuis TJ. Neutrophils contribute to fracture healing by synthesizing fibronectin+ extracellular matrix rapidly after injury. Clinical Immunology. 2016 **164**:78-84

[114] Kovtun A, Bergdolt S, Wiegner R, Radermacher P, Huber-Lang M, Ignatius A. The crucial role of neutrophil granulocytes in bone fracture healing. European Cells & Materials. 2016;**32**: 152-162

[115] Chakravarti A, Raquil MA, Tessier P, Poubelle PE. Surface RANKL of Toll-like receptor 4-stimulated human neutrophils activates osteoclastic bone resorption. Blood. 2009;**114**(8): 1633-1644

[116] Quinn JM, Neale S, Fujikawa Y, McGee JO, Athanasou NA. Human osteoclast formation from blood monocytes, peritoneal macrophages, and bone marrow cells. Calcified Tissue International. 1998;**62**(6):527-531

[117] Sugisaki R, Miyamoto Y, Yoshimura K, Sasa K, Kaneko K, Tanaka M, et al. Possible involvement of elastase in enhanced osteoclast differentiation by neutrophils through degradation of osteoprotegerin. Bone. 2020;**132**:115216

[118] Moutsopoulos NM, Konkel J, Sarmadi M, Eskan MA, Wild T, Dutzan N, et al. Defective neutrophil recruitment in leukocyte adhesion deficiency type I disease causes local IL-17-driven inflammatory bone loss. Science Translational Medicine. 2014; **6**(229):229ra40

[119] Blom AB, van Lent PL, Holthuysen AE, van der Kraan PM, Roth J, van Rooijen N, et al. Synovial lining macrophages mediate osteophyte formation during experimental

osteoarthritis. Osteoarthritis and Cartilage. 2004;**12**(8):627-635

[120] Chang MK, Raggatt LJ, Alexander KA, Kuliwaba JS, Fazzalari NL, Schroder K, et al. Osteal tissue macrophages are intercalated throughout human and mouse bone lining tissues and regulate osteoblast function in vitro and in vivo. Journal of Immunology. 2008;**181**(2):1232-1244

[121] Murray PJ, Allen JE, Biswas SK, Fisher EA, Gilroy DW, Goerdt S, et al. Macrophage activation and polarization: Nomenclature and experimental guidelines. Immunity. 2014;**41**(1):14-20

[122] Lassus J, Salo J, Jiranek WA, Santavirta S, Nevalainen J, Matucci-Cerinic M, et al. Macrophage activation results in bone resorption. Clinical Orthopaedics and Related Research. 1998;**352**:7-15

[123] Yamaguchi T, Movila A, Kataoka S, Wisitrasameewong W, Ruiz Torruella M, Murakoshi M, et al. Proinflammatory M1 macrophages inhibit RANKL-induced osteoclastogenesis. Infection and Immunity. 2016;**84**(10):2802-2812

[124] Huang R, Wang X, Zhou Y, Xiao Y. RANKL-induced M1 macrophages are involved in bone formation. Bone Research. 2017;**5**:17019

[125] Schlundt C, El Khassawna T, Serra A, Dienelt A, Wendler S, Schell H, et al. Macrophages in bone fracture healing: Their essential role in endochondral ossification. Bone. 2018;**106**:78-89

[126] Dou C, Ding N, Zhao C, Hou T, Kang F, Cao Z, et al. Estrogen deficiency-mediated M2 macrophage osteoclastogenesis contributes to M1/M2 ratio alteration in ovariectomized osteoporotic mice. Journal of Bone and Mineral Research. 2018;**33**(5):899-908

[127] Gallois A, Lachuer J, Yvert G, Wierinckx A, Brunet F, Rabourdin-Combe C, et al. Genome-wide expression analyses establish dendritic cells as a new osteoclast precursor able to generate bone-resorbing cells more efficiently than monocytes. Journal of Bone and Mineral Research. 2010;**25**(3):661-672

[128] Santiago-Schwarz F, Anand P, Liu S, Carsons SE. Dendritic cells (DCs) in rheumatoid arthritis (RA): Progenitor cells and soluble factors contained in RA synovial fluid yield a subset of myeloid DCs that preferentially activate Th1 inflammatory-type responses. Journal of Immunology. 2001;**167**(3):1758-1768

[129] Rivollier A, Mazzorana M, Tebib J, Piperno M, Aitsiselmi T, Rabourdin-Combe C, et al. Immature dendritic cell transdifferentiation into osteoclasts: A novel pathway sustained by the rheumatoid arthritis microenvironment. Blood. 2004;**104**(13):4029-4037

[130] Cline-Smith A, Axelbaum A, Shashkova E, Chakraborty M, Sanford J, Panesar P, et al. Ovariectomy activates chronic low-grade inflammation mediated by memory T cells, which promotes osteoporosis in mice. Journal of Bone and Mineral Research. 2020;**35**(6):1174-1187

[131] Takayanagi H, Ogasawara K, Hida S, Chiba T, Murata S, Sato K, et al. T-cell-mediated regulation of osteoclastogenesis by signalling cross-talk between RANKL and IFN-gamma. Nature. 2000;**408**(6812):600-605

[132] Jin Y, Wi HJ, Choi MH, Hong ST, Bae YM. Regulation of anti-inflammatory cytokines IL-10 and TGF-beta in mouse dendritic cells

through treatment with Clonorchis sinensis crude antigen. Experimental & Molecular Medicine. 2014;**46**(1):e74

[133] Onal M, Xiong J, Chen X, Thostenson JD, Almeida M, Manolagas SC, et al. Receptor activator of nuclear factor kappaB ligand (RANKL) protein expression by B lymphocytes contributes to ovariectomy-induced bone loss. The Journal of Biological Chemistry. 2012; **287**(35):29851-29860

[134] Sun W, Meednu N, Rosenberg A, Rangel-Moreno J, Wang V, Glanzman J, et al. B cells inhibit bone formation in rheumatoid arthritis by suppressing osteoblast differentiation. Nature Communications. 2018;**9**(1):5127

[135] Fujiwara Y, Piemontese M, Liu Y, Thostenson JD, Xiong J, O'Brien CA. RANKL (receptor activator of NFkappaB ligand) produced by osteocytes is required for the increase in B cells and bone loss caused by estrogen deficiency in mice. The Journal of Biological Chemistry. 2016;**291**(48):24838-24850

[136] Konnecke I, Serra A, El Khassawna T, Schlundt C, Schell H, Hauser A, et al. T and B cells participate in bone repair by infiltrating the fracture callus in a two-wave fashion. Bone. 2014; **64**:155-165

[137] Hughes DE, Dai A, Tiffee JC, Li HH, Mundy GR, Boyce BF. Estrogen promotes apoptosis of murine osteoclasts mediated by TGF-beta. Nature Medicine. 1996;**2**(10):1132-1136

[138] Sapra L, Bhardwaj A, Mishra PK, Garg B, Verma B, Mishra GC, et al. Regulatory B cells (Bregs) inhibit osteoclastogenesis and play a potential role in ameliorating ovariectomy-induced bone loss. Frontiers in Immunology. 2021;**12**:691081

[139] Srivastava RK, Sapra L. The rising era of "Immunoporosis": Role of immune system in the pathophysiology of osteoporosis. Journal of Inflammation Research. 2022;**15**:1667-1698

[140] Choi Y, Woo KM, Ko SH, Lee YJ, Park SJ, Kim HM, et al. Osteoclastogenesis is enhanced by activated B cells but suppressed by activated CD8(+) T cells. European Journal of Immunology. 2001;**31**(7): 2179-2188

[141] Terauchi M, Li JY, Bedi B, Baek KH, Tawfeek H, Galley S, et al. T lymphocytes amplify the anabolic activity of parathyroid hormone through Wnt10b signaling. Cell Metabolism. 2009;**10**(3):229-240

[142] Bedi B, Li JY, Tawfeek H, Baek KH, Adams J, Vangara SS, et al. Silencing of parathyroid hormone (PTH) receptor 1 in T cells blunts the bone anabolic activity of PTH. Proceedings of the National Academy of Sciences of the United States of America. 2012;**109**(12): E725-E733

[143] Yamada A, Takami M, Kawawa T, Yasuhara R, Zhao B, Mochizuki A, et al. Interleukin-4 inhibition of osteoclast differentiation is stronger than that of interleukin-13 and they are equivalent for induction of osteoprotegerin production from osteoblasts. Immunology. 2007;**120**(4):573-579

[144] Gao Y, Grassi F, Ryan MR, Terauchi M, Page K, Yang X, et al. IFN-gamma stimulates osteoclast formation and bone loss in vivo via antigen-driven T cell activation. The Journal of Clinical Investigation. 2007;**117**(1):122-132

[145] Noonan K, Marchionni L, Anderson J, Pardoll D, Roodman GD, Borrello I. A novel role of IL-17-producing lymphocytes in mediating

lytic bone disease in multiple myeloma. Blood. 2010;**116**(18):3554-3563

[146] Lei H, Schmidt-Bleek K, Dienelt A, Reinke P, Volk HD. Regulatory T cell-mediated anti-inflammatory effects promote successful tissue repair in both indirect and direct manners. Frontiers in Pharmacology. 2015;**6**:184

[147] Tyagi AM, Yu M, Darby TM, Vaccaro C, Li JY, Owens JA, et al. The microbial metabolite butyrate stimulates bone formation via T regulatory cell-mediated regulation of WNT10B expression. Immunity. 2018;**49**(6): 1116-31 e7

[148] Kar S, Gupta R, Malhotra R, Sharma V, Farooque K, Kumar V, et al. Interleukin-9 facilitates osteoclastogenesis in rheumatoid arthritis. International Journal of Molecular Sciences. 2021;**22**(19):10397

[149] Monasterio G, Budini V, Fernandez B, Castillo F, Rojas C, Alvarez C, et al. IL-22-expressing CD4 (+) AhR(+) T lymphocytes are associated with RANKL-mediated alveolar bone resorption during experimental periodontitis. Journal of Periodontal Research. 2019;**54**(5): 513-524

[150] Xu F, Li W, Yang X, Na L, Chen L, Liu G. The roles of epigenetics regulation in bone metabolism and osteoporosis. Frontiers in Cell and Development Biology. 2020;**8**:619301

[151] Kiselev IS, Kulakova OG, Boyko AN, Favorova OO. DNA methylation As an epigenetic mechanism in the development of multiple sclerosis. Acta Naturae. 2021;**13**(2):45-57

[152] Alaskhar Alhamwe B, Khalaila R, Wolf J, von Bulow V, Harb H, Alhamdan F, et al. Histone modifications and their role in epigenetics of atopy and allergic diseases. Allergy, Asthma and Clinical Immunology. 2018;**14**:39

[153] Biswas S, Rao CM. Epigenetic tools (the writers, the readers and the erasers) and their implications in cancer therapy. European Journal of Pharmacology. 2018;**837**:8-24

[154] Zhang P, Liu Y, Jin C, Zhang M, Lv L, Zhang X, et al. Histone H3K9 acetyltransferase PCAF is essential for osteogenic differentiation through bone morphogenetic protein signaling and may Be involved in osteoporosis. Stem Cells. 2016;**34**(9):2332-2341

[155] Kim S, Shevde NK, Pike JW. 1,25-Dihydroxyvitamin D3 stimulates cyclic vitamin D receptor/retinoid X receptor DNA-binding, co-activator recruitment, and histone acetylation in intact osteoblasts. Journal of Bone and Mineral Research. 2005;**20**(2):305-317

[156] Meyer MB, Benkusky NA, Sen B, Rubin J, Pike JW. Epigenetic plasticity drives adipogenic and osteogenic differentiation of marrow-derived mesenchymal stem cells. The Journal of Biological Chemistry. 2016;**291**(34): 17829-17847

[157] Meier JC, Tallant C, Fedorov O, Witwicka H, Hwang SY, van Stiphout RG, et al. Selective targeting of bromodomains of the bromodomain-PHD fingers family impairs osteoclast differentiation. ACS Chemical Biology. 2017;**12**(10):2619-2630

[158] Yi SJ, Lee H, Lee J, Lee K, Kim J, Kim Y, et al. Bone remodeling: Histone modifications as fate determinants of bone cell differentiation. International Journal of Molecular Sciences. 2019;**20**(13):3147

[159] Lee HW, Suh JH, Kim AY, Lee YS, Park SY, Kim JB. Histone deacetylase

1-mediated histone modification regulates osteoblast differentiation. Molecular Endocrinology. 2006;**20**(10): 2432-2443

[160] Feigenson M, Shull LC, Taylor EL, Camilleri ET, Riester SM, van Wijnen AJ, et al. Histone deacetylase 3 deletion in mesenchymal progenitor cells hinders long bone development. Journal of Bone and Mineral Research. 2017; **32**(12):2453-2465

[161] Hakelien AM, Bryne JC, Harstad KG, Lorenz S, Paulsen J, Sun J, et al. The regulatory landscape of osteogenic differentiation. Stem Cells. 2014;**32**(10):2780-2793

[162] Hemming S, Cakouros D, Isenmann S, Cooper L, Menicanin D, Zannettino A, et al. EZH2 and KDM6A act as an epigenetic switch to regulate mesenchymal stem cell lineage specification. Stem Cells. 2014;**32**(3): 802-815

[163] Kota SK, Roening C, Patel N, Kota SB, Baron R. PRMT5 inhibition promotes osteogenic differentiation of mesenchymal stromal cells and represses basal interferon stimulated gene expression. Bone. 2018;**117**:37-46

[164] Fang C, Qiao Y, Mun SH, Lee MJ, Murata K, Bae S, et al. Cutting edge: EZH2 promotes osteoclastogenesis by epigenetic silencing of the negative regulator IRF8. Journal of Immunology. 2016;**196**(11):4452-4456

[165] Gao Y, Ge W. The histone methyltransferase DOT1L inhibits osteoclastogenesis and protects against osteoporosis. Cell Death & Disease. 2018;**9**(2):33

[166] Ohguchi H, Harada T, Sagawa M, Kikuchi S, Tai YT, Richardson PG, et al. KDM6B modulates MAPK pathway mediating multiple myeloma cell growth and survival. Leukemia. 2017;**31**(12): 2661-2669

[167] Yang D, Okamura H, Nakashima Y, Haneji T. Histone demethylase Jmjd3 regulates osteoblast differentiation via transcription factors Runx2 and osterix. The Journal of Biological Chemistry. 2013;**288**(47):33530-33541

[168] Rojas A, Aguilar R, Henriquez B, Lian JB, Stein JL, Stein GS, et al. Epigenetic control of the bone-master Runx2 gene during osteoblast-lineage commitment by the histone demethylase JARID1B/KDM5B. The Journal of Biological Chemistry. 2015;**290**(47): 28329-28342